Praise for *The TMJ Handbook*

"Cator Shachoy offers three beautifully aligned, complimentary entry points to healing from TMD—bodywork, yoga, and mindfulness meditation. And she gently and confidently supports her healing program on the two palms of compassion and kindness." —Allison Post, coauthor of *Unwinding the Belly*

"Cator Shachoy's contribution to the treatment of TMD is easy to follow, even for those without a background in anatomy and yoga. I know that the exercises and meditations will bring positive results for TMD—and for the body and mind." —Benjamin Shield, PhD, coauthor of *Handbook for the Soul*

"A thoroughly empowering guide to bring a new holistic perspective and treatment to a challenging, often overlooked issue" —Christopher Willard, PsyD, author of *Growing Up Mindful*

"To my knowledge, this is the first book that deals exclusively and at length with TMJ disorders and their relief. Cator Shachoy first lays the groundwork by looking at the many causes of the condition, then goes on to suggest a variety of treatments including breath work, self-massage, mindfulness, and yoga-based exercises. This is a well-rounded, fully accessible, intelligently organized program that should prove highly effective in the self-treatment of TMD." —Richard Rosen, author of *Yoga by the Numbers*

"I highly recommend Cator's book for anyone interested in working with their jaw/TMJ tension and body tension in general." —Franklyn Sills, BCST, author of *Foundations in Craniosacral Biodynamics* vols 1 and 2

"*The TMJ Handbook* provides deep and tangible jewels of insight to both patients and experts. A must-have for longtime jaw tension sufferers."
—Holly Edson, NP, Craniosacral Therapist

"Drawing on decades of practice in mindfulness and yoga, Cator Shachoy guides us with clarity, simple exercises, and a friendly approach to let go of the unconscious causes of jaw tension (TMD). Of course, jaw tension isn't just about the jaw—this is a manual for body and mind." —Anandabodhi Bhikkuni, abbess, Aloka Vihara

"Cator Shachoy takes relieving jaw tension as a starting point but then expands to include our human experience. There is a broad approach to cultivating mindfulness and body awareness along with tips on how to include all this in daily life. This book is immensely practical as well as clear, coherent, and down-to-earth." —Pasanno Bhikkhu, former abbot, Abhyagiri Buddhist Monastery

"This book will be enlightening for anyone who suffers from jaw tension as well as bodyworkers and therapists who want to learn more. I highly recommend *The TMJ Handbook*—it will help so many people!" —Deborah Wolk, founder of Samamkaya Yoga Back Care & Scoliosis Collective NYC

"*The TMJ Handbook* is an exceptional contribution to the field of health, and essential reading for all concerned with reducing stress and increasing well-being."—Thanissara, author of *Time to Stand Up*

The TMJ Handbook

A Therapeutic Guide to Relieving Jaw Tension and Pain with Yoga and Mindfulness

Cator Shachoy

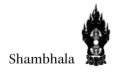

Shambhala

Shambhala Publications, Inc.
2129 13th Street
Boulder, Colorado 80302
www.shambhala.com

9 8 7 6 5 4 3 2 1

First Edition
Printed in the United States of America

Shambhala Publications makes every effort to print on acid-free, recycled paper.
Shambhala Publications is distributed worldwide by Penguin Random House, Inc.,
and its subsidiaries.

Library of Congress Cataloging-in-Publication Data
Names: Shachoy, Cator, author.
Title: The TMJ handbook: a therapeutic guide to relieving jaw tension
and pain with yoga and mindfulness / Cator Shachoy.
Other titles: Temporomandibular joint handbook
Description: Boulder, Colorado: Shambhala Publications, Inc., [2024] |
Includes bibliographical references and index.
Identifiers: LCCN 2022011533 | ISBN 9781645471035 (trade paperback)
Subjects: LCSH: Temporomandibular joint—Diseases—Exercise therapy—
Handbooks, manuals, etc.—Popular works. | Temporomandibular joint—
Diseases—Prevention—Handbooks, manuals, etc.—Popular works.
Classification: LCC RK470 .S48 2022 | DDC 617.5/220624—dc23/eng/20220318
LC record available at https://lccn.loc.gov/2022011533

Dedication

To my one and only mom,
Mollie Jenckes
who has always stood by me,
even when my choices were unusual

To my teachers
who have guided me with patience,
kindness and forgiveness

To my students and clients
who inspire and teach me

To my friends who accept me with all my foibles,
provide companionship
and more than a little fun along the way

Contents

PART THREE: Mindfulness Exercises

Audio recordings of Guided Meditations are available
for free download at www.catorshachoy.com.

List of Figures

Foreword

O VER THE YEARS of Cator Shachoy's practice and teaching she received repeated requests for guidance and advice concerning problems of jaw tension. This is the source of why Cator has written *The TMJ Handbook: A Therapeutic Guide to Relieving Jaw Tension and Pain with Yoga and Mindfulness* as a comprehensive book using relief of jaw tension as the basis. With Cator's extensive background in yoga, craniosacral bodywork, and mindfulness training, she is covering many bases to give the reader tools to work on themselves physically and for reflection and contemplation.

Cator does an excellent job in addressing the reality that our bodies and minds are not discrete entities but rather complexly woven together, interacting and affecting each other in many ways. She takes us on a journey of the body through the anatomy of how the jaw affects, and is affected by, the rest of our body. There are physical practices that are detailed in order to have the tools for helping ourselves. Plus, there are investigations suggested throughout that will help to create a sense of perspective supportive of better understanding of our human condition. This is a handbook or a tool kit for working on ourselves.

I have known Cator Shachoy now for over twenty-five years and have seen her search, practice, question, and train herself so that she is able to speak confidently from her own experience. She has taught and helped others for a long time, and the skills she has gained from this service are made manifest in this book. It is a delight to see her knowledge become something solid on the page of a book. I hope that this book fulfills her intention of helping others to experience ease, well-being, and clarity.

Ajahn Pasanno, resident elder and former abbot,
Abhayagiri Buddhist Monastery, Redwood Valley, California

Acknowledgments

THIS PROJECT has taken a bit of time to manifest—about eight years to be exact. However, the time it has taken has allowed it to stew and marinate in the best of ways, generating a far richer and heartier broth than might have happened otherwise. I am deeply grateful to the kind and generous support of so many people, far more than I can name or personally thank and not the least of which includes the many students and clients who have sought me out and invited me into their experience. I have learned so much from your personal journeys. I bow in gratitude for the opportunity to be of service and continue to grow through the relationships that result from offering this beautiful work.

I want to thank Ajahn Pasanno, Ayya Anandabodhi, Benjamin Shield, Franklyn Sills, Richard Rosen, and Ryan Halford for willingly reading through the manuscript at different stages, thus providing an invaluable service. Thank you to Benjamin Shield, Ellen Mossman, Franklyn Sills, Hugh Milne, and Ryan Halford for letting me pick their brains on different subjects related to this book. Ruth Denison, an extraordinary person and meditation teacher, taught oral cavity guided meditations extending for an hour or more that were so engrossing they inspired me to include the practice in my workshops, albeit more briefly. Several volunteers helped to work through the anatomy section. In writing this chapter I found out there are two types of people in the world: those who find anatomy interesting, exciting, and even thrilling; and those who will be significantly happier if the subject is never broached again. As you might imagine, myself and many of my friends and colleagues are in the former group (my fellow somanauts!), while my developmental editor turned out to be in the latter group. Ultimately this was a gift. With the intention to make this chapter more accessible, I reached out to a wider circle of readers. The final result is intended to be inviting to those who don't care for anatomy while still interesting and informative to the somanauts. Thanks to Aleksandra Kumorek, Dawn Richards, Ellen Mossman, Mollie Jenckes, Stephen Schiller, Susan Morgan, and Thomas Sprenkle. My writing buddy Susan Morgan kept the project moving forward through our monthly phone calls and annual writing retreats.

In addition to reading the anatomy section, Mollie Jenckes is a nurse and public health researcher for Johns Hopkins University and also happens to be my mother. She has offered her generous support in many ways. I was visiting her home in Baltimore, Maryland, when pandemic restrictions were put in place nationwide in early March 2020. And there I remained for six months. While this was unexpected for both of us, it ended up offering the chance to work on this manuscript. I remain grateful for our days together, a special time with my one and only mom. Eventually Catherine Byers invited me to stay in San Carlos, and so I returned to California. Her generosity allowed me to finish this project. Catherine and Amanda Kovattana offered a supportive environment through open ears and hearts and providing feedback. I couldn't have landed in a better place. The pandemic proved the perfect opportunity to git 'er done.

Developmental editor Kim Criswell has been an essential crutch for me to lean on. This was a far larger project than I had previously attempted, and her organizational skills were a wonderful asset. The team of Denise Matsubara Lapidus, Dina Hondrogen, Eva Enriquez, and Jenny Schaffer helped with the yoga and core actions photographs that were used to create illustrations. Shambhala editor Beth Frankl with her grace and skill has gently guided me in the process of publication. And art director Lora Zorian's expertise was a huge asset with regard to putting the book together. The entire Shambhala team has been amazing. There are many more unseen hands and hearts who have contributed to the book you hold in your hands (or read on a screen). I bow to each and every one of you for your contributions to this project.

I have been incredibly lucky to train and study with exceptional teachers over the past thirty years, many of whom have inspired aspects of this book. I have tried to convey information with veracity and integrity. Any inaccuracies that remain are mine alone. I invite you to take what is useful and leave the rest behind.

> May all beings be safe, happy, protected, and at ease.
> May we all live in peace together.
>
> —Cator Shachoy

Disclaimer

The information and practices offered in this book are not a substitute for medical advice. Please consult a doctor to see whether yoga and/or mindfulness are appropriate for you. Stop any practice that causes discomfort or distress and seek appropriate support for the condition. All names have been changed when referring to client stories. The stories portrayed are inspired by client interactions; they do not reflect a single individual, but rather represent an amalgam of experience.

Introduction

THE BODY OF WORK presented in this book came directly out of my experience teaching yoga and mindfulness classes, workshops, and retreats publicly, as well as my private practice as a craniosacral bodyworker, yoga therapist, and mindfulness guide. As a cranial practitioner I have worked with many people with jaw tension. For those unfamiliar with craniosacral, it is a very gentle, effective health care modality involving specific touch with light pressure. My practice is in San Francisco, California, where a large portion of my clients are familiar with yoga and mindfulness. Thus it was completely natural for me to suggest yoga poses and mindfulness practices for those interested in learning how to help themselves recover from chronic or acute jaw tension.

In working with people's bodies, I have observed a relationship between their breathing and jaw tension. In response I often suggested breathing exercises to support greater health. Over time I noticed that people began to unravel the habit of clenching and grinding through cultivating self-awareness. Seeing this encouraged me to train people in mindfulness and loving-kindness practices so that they could become more aware of their habits and learn for themselves the causes of tension. Mindfulness gives us a way of seeing cause and effect in our own bodies and minds. Loving-kindness provides a means for holding what we see with compassionate awareness. We need to be very gentle with ourselves as we begin to heal old patterns.

The yoga poses presented in this book are informed by an understanding that is unique to craniosacral therapy regarding how your jaw interacts with the rest of your body. If we think about it a little, it makes perfect sense that your jaw is a part of your whole body and thus receptive to influences from just about anywhere. There are pluses and minuses to this—but ultimately this book makes positive use of this information, engaging whole body yoga poses to beneficially realign your jaw. Craniosacral bodywork has a very refined and sophisticated understanding of the human jaw—unlike anything I have experienced anywhere else. This uncommon view is rooted in understanding originally developed by Dr. William Sutherland and others in the early 1900s and has been verified by thousands of practitioners in private practice over more than one hundred years. This is a body of work developed through direct experience born out of the client-practitioner relationship and then further distilled via communication among cranial therapists around the world as they sought to polish techniques and develop protocols that bring effective relief.

Mindfulness, loving-kindness, and compassion practices are essential influences on this body of work as well. I began teaching a weekly yoga and meditation class at the Zen Hospice Project in San Francisco in 2002. The class was open to the general public and continued for ten years. The benefits of incorporating mindfulness practice with yoga were apparent immediately and grew over time. Participants enjoyed the opportunity for quiet and cultivated greater self-awareness regarding their habits of mind and body.

Meanwhile, in my private practice, I found that many people were receptive to learning how they can help themselves heal. While it takes effort and is not always easy, we can learn how to care for ourselves in body and mind through the practice of mindful awareness. This simple, self-reflective practice can be applied to our daily actions and provides a means for unraveling unconscious tendencies that may initially seem innocuous. Over time, through reflection, we begin to see the destructive aspects of these habits. Upon becoming aware, our wisdom mind invites us to let go. Loving-kindness and compassion are essential in this process. These qualities of mind teach us how to hold both ourselves and others. Rather than indulging a self-critical, judgmental, or defensive attitude, we can train ourselves to relate from a place of compassion, learning to cultivate a quality of friendship toward ourselves and others. This is a requisite component in healing—for ourselves, our primary relationships, our community, and the planet.

I have several intentions in making this body of work available to the general public. The first is to educate people on the causes and repercussions of jaw tension from the cranial perspective. The information available through craniosacral therapy is not only accurate but also rare and fascinating—

and not generally available in our culture due to the structure of our current health care system. This unavailability in no way invalidates this body of work. In fact, my experience of teaching the Yoga for Jaw Tension workshop over sixty times since 2011 demonstrates there is a tremendous need for this information. It is extremely helpful to those who suffer from jaw tension, as well as your average somanaut looking to better understand interactions between physiology and brain. Craniosacral bodywork recognizes and clearly explains cross-connections throughout the body not understood by the conventional allopathic medical model.

Through the cranial model we can understand that the causes of jaw tension are wide-ranging, including car accidents, whiplash, blows to the head or neck, other physical trauma, as well as dental work, braces, expanders, and other dental interventions. All forms of trauma and societal isms can be factors. Jaw tension can also be caused by birth. There can be many years between the original trauma and onset of symptoms—even twenty years or more. Physical and emotional traumas that remain unresolved continue to influence the tissues, over time resulting in significant tension.

Likewise, the repercussions of jaw tension are widespread, including pain when biting or chewing, clicking or popping in the jaw, and jaw muscles that are painful or sore to the touch. For many, chronic jaw tension includes the habit of grinding their teeth while sleeping. This can mean waking up with pain in the face, a tight or sore neck and shoulders, and sometimes headaches—including migraines. Being unable to fully open your mouth or bite into hard foods can be a part of jaw tension. Broken crowns, worn-down teeth, root canals, sinus infections, and ringing in the ears can also go along with jaw tension. Other issues that can be associated include tight hips, groin muscles, and psoas, as well as digestive disorders and, for women, menstrual or hormonal disorders. Part one of this book—Jaw Tension Explained—will explain how this is possible.

All of the material in this book has been tested out first in my private practice, then through public classes and workshops. In addition to providing conceptual information, I offer a range of tools for helping yourself. A variety of self-care practices are presented because there are a variety of people and personalities on the planet and different approaches appeal to different people. There are many resources detailed in this book. In part one—Jaw Tension Explained—we discuss face and jaw self-massage and an introduction to conscious touch (see chapter 8). In part two—Yoga for Relief—you will find simple postural awareness techniques called Core Actions (chapter 10) as well as yoga postures (chapter 11) and sequences for practitioners at various levels (chapter 12). Part three—Mindfulness Exercises—details breathing exercises, guided meditations, and mindfulness practices to round out a complete program. Additionally, audio recordings of the guided meditations are available for free download at www.catorshachoy.com. Hopefully most people will find something that is useful to them—and possibly several things.

The techniques shared here focus on building self-awareness so that you can learn more about your personal tension patterns and what brings you relief. The more attuned we can become to our habits of stress, the quicker we will be able to change these inclinations and unravel tension. Over time we then start noticing the tension or stressor sooner. This allows us to address it more quickly. Simultaneously, we are unlearning the habit of our stress response, cultivating greater stability and ease.

Self-awareness skills can be used for a variety of issues—not just jaw tension. In most, if not all, cases these tools will benefit your life even after your jaw tension is resolved. They are in no way harmful, but rather generally beneficial, so it's a win-win. In this regard I would like to introduce the principle of *ehipassiko*. Translated as "encouraging investigation" or "come and see for yourself," this word was used by the Buddha again and again as an exhortation to *trust your own deepest experience*. His intention was to encourage each of us to not simply take his—or anyone else's—word as truth. Instead, he invited us to cultivate mindful awareness and really know our own experience. You can know the answers to many things simply through paying attention. In this light, the principle of ehipassiko underlies this body of work. Don't simply take my word for it, but rather, give it a try. See whether it works for you.

Lastly, my hope in making this body of work available to you is that it will empower and motivate you to become an active participant in your own health and well-being. This book provides numerous simple ways to consider how you can help yourself to live life with less pain and distress while simultaneously feeling more at ease, peaceful, happy, connected, and a part of the world around you on a daily basis. I invite you to view caring for your body and mind as a way to get to know yourself better. Your careful attention to your well-being can be an expression of your heart. Let it become an opportunity to fall in love with yourself—and everyone around you. And don't forget to enjoy the journey!

PART ONE
Jaw Tension Explained

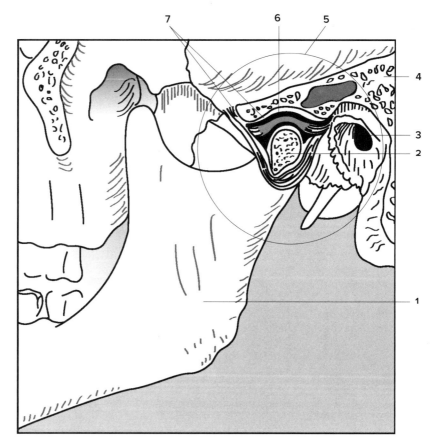

Figure 1.1: Anatomy of the TMJ. This illustration shows the inner workings of the temporomandibular joint.

1. mandible
2. condyle (outer portion removed)
3. ear canal
4. temporal bone

5. TMJ
6. disc
7. synovial spaces

❧ 1

Jaw Tension Defined: TMJ vs. TMD

WHAT IS *TMD* and how is it different from *TMJ*? Let's a take a closer look at your jaw to better understand. TMJ stands for *temporomandibular joint*. This is the joint that connects the bone of your ear, or *temporal*, and your lower jawbone, or *mandible*, allowing you to open and close your mouth. Everyone has two TMJs located on either side of their head, just below and in front of their ears. It is important to distinguish between the joint itself—the temporomandibular joint—and the condition of jaw tension. **In this book, *TMJ* refers only to the joint.** *TMD*—**temporomandibular joint dysfunction—refers to the condition of an imbalanced and painful jaw or joint. The term** *jaw tension* **is used synonymously with** *TMD*.

Who Suffers from TMD?

It's difficult to find accurate statistics regarding TMD. Definitions of the condition vary and can impact reported cases. *Netter's Head and Neck Anatomy for Dentists* states that 33 percent of adults[1] have chronic jaw tension—that means over 110 million people in 2023. And that's just in the United States. While all genders are affected, women are at least twice as likely to experience TMD.[2] Health professionals long believed women ages twenty to forty were most affected. However, recent research reviewing TMD in the United States and Europe indicates it peaks much later, between ages forty-six to sixty-four.[3] The age at which TMD is most common brings up questions regarding a possible link with hormones, in particular estrogen. At the same time, prevalence in youth ages ten to nineteen years old is between 7 and

30 percent.[4] What all of this tells us is TMD can in fact occur at almost any age—from very young to elderly. It is a universal health condition around the globe.

An experience I had after teaching a yoga class gives us some idea of just how pervasive TMD is. During my weekly yoga and meditation class I decided to focus on jaw tension and ways to work with it that can provide relief. The program wasn't announced in advance, so participants weren't aware of the subject matter ahead of time. Afterward, a young woman came up to ask a question. We stood and talked while everyone gathered their belongings to clear the space. Before we had finished our conversation, I noticed that *every woman* who had attended had joined us to contribute an anecdote about their own struggle with a tight or painful jaw.

Understanding TMD

A surprising range of physical conditions can be linked to jaw tension. TMD often results from a variety of conditions coming together and may take many years to manifest. Clenching and grinding your teeth can result in cracked and broken teeth, caps, crowns, root canals, and tooth replacement. Dental work, such as braces, expanders, poorly fitted bridges, fillings, extractions, filed teeth, and other interventions can also be a *cause* of jaw tension.

Sometimes sinusitis, ear infections, hearing sensitivity or loss, inner ear disorders, and tinnitus (ringing in the ears) are associated with TMD. All manner of headaches including tension, cluster, and migraine, as well as stiff or frozen shoulders, scoliosis, lower back pain, sacroiliac imbalance, tight psoas or groin muscles, and sciatica can be linked to imbalanced or tight TMJs. Hormonal and menstrual disorders as well as poor digestion can be connected to jaw tension. In fact, TMD can extend down into the knees and feet, even causing bunions. Strange though it may seem, jaw tension can have an impact from the top of your head down to the tips of your toes. We'll explore how this is possible throughout part one.

Physical trauma such as car accidents, sports injuries (think skiing, biking, or running), as well as slip and fall mishaps can result in jaw tension, even when the jaw does not appear to be directly involved. In addition to physical factors, TMD can be tied to psychological issues. Emotional trauma and stress are factors in jaw tension. How do we survive situations we are uncomfortable with or don't want? The many cultural references to jaw tension come to mind: *Grit your teeth and bear it. Bite your tongue. Chew on that. A tough pill to swallow.*

Something as common as being called names as a child or criticized in front of our peers can make us clench. Or maybe you were jumped in a dark alleyway or coerced in other ways by people close to you. Perhaps your personal sense of integrity was violated in less overt, more covert ways by people in your life or by society in general—systemic sexism, racism, and other isms can contribute to jaw tension. The habit of clenching or grinding may show up right away or many years after trauma occurs. What causes us to clench is often a combination of physical, emotional, psychological, and/or systemic trauma.

And, finally, even birth itself can lay a foundation for TMD to manifest as we mature into adulthood. Birthing dynamics are complex, with intense forces involved through the combination of contractions and positioning. An infant's skull needs to become exactly the size of the mother's pelvis to emerge. This means skull bones will overlap during birthing. A baby's head generally resets itself during the first few days after being born. However, imbalances in the skull can remain.[5] While C-section births may appear to be gentler, they can also impact the head and jaw.

Night Guards—Help or Harm?

The most common treatment for TMD at this time is a night guard—a dentist-prescribed splint worn at night to mitigate repercussions from clenching and grinding during sleep. I am frequently asked whether they help or not. If you wake up to find your night guard in the far corner of your room because you (un)wittingly tossed it there at some point during the night, you are not alone. It's fairly common for clients to express dislike for and distrust in the efficacy of this approach—not to mention it can be very expensive, uncomfortable, and yes, unflattering to put a piece of plastic in your mouth in front of your partner before going to bed each night.

Still, a well-fitted night guard can help in a few ways. It will keep you from wearing down the biting surface of your teeth. This is important. Your teeth need to last a long time. We each get just two sets of teeth, and the first is gone by age thirteen. The wear of grinding your teeth at night (bruxism) can result in cracked or broken teeth and the need for caps, crowns, bridges, or tooth replacement, as well as root canals, sinus infections, and tinnitus, among other issues. The process necessary for all of this dental work is costly, time-consuming, and potentially traumatic.

The appropriate dental device can also mitigate symptoms related to clenching. Since there is a forced separation between your teeth, muscles cannot contract as tightly, which can reduce headaches, neck and shoulder aches, and pain in the teeth and face. Additionally, a splint can protect the TMJs from further damage. Clenching can literally destroy your jaw joint—overextending ligaments, rupturing the disc, changing the shape of the bone itself—which leads to discomfort, difficulty biting and chewing, and other painful conditions.

It's worth noting that a poorly fitted device or an over-the-counter version may cause harm through misalignment of mouth, jaw, face, and neck. If symptoms increase after using a device, stop using it. If the prescribed night guard developed by your dentist is not offering relief, it is worthwhile to contact them and make sure it is fitting well and possibly explore a different model of splint. Do research, find out which dentist in your area specializes in TMD, and consider giving them a call. A second opinion or switch of practitioner may be worthwhile.

It is important to recognize that a night guard does not stop the habit of clenching and grinding. It is a symptomatic treatment, not a cure. Thus, it can help you feel better on a daily basis but will not be the same as solving the original cause of the problem. The night guard does not get to the root question of *why do I do this?*

That is where this book comes in. *You can resolve this habit.* You can find answers to the question *why?* through investigating cause and effect. In the chapters that follow, we will look at the contributing factors to jaw tension through a variety of lenses. We will then examine *how* to unravel this painful and destructive habit using a range of self-care practices as tools.

EXERCISE: NOTICE HOW YOUR JAW WORKS

The best way to understand jaw tension is to investigate it directly. In the introduction I mentioned the principle of ehipassiko or *trusting your own experience*. I encourage you to go back to this again and again. Let's take a moment to check out how your jaw is working today, from the inside out. Try this exercise. Open and close your mouth a few times while looking in a mirror. Which side of your mouth opens more fully? Does your lower lip pull to the right or left? Listen closely for clicking, grinding, or popping in your jaw. What about your ears, do they pop? Is it painful to open or close your mouth? Does one side hurt more than the other? (This exercise is included with greater detail in chapter 15; see page 207.)

By investigating what happens with your jaw when you open and close it you can begin to understand imbalances in your TMJs more directly. This lays a foundation for relieving tension. A question to consider is, *at what point does jaw tension cause discomfort and begin to negatively impact your lifestyle, health, and well-being?*

Jaw tension is a fascinating condition with many influences—physical alignment, body structure, personal life experience, as well as cultural and societal factors. In the chapters that follow, we'll look at the complex web of interconnections between your jaw, the rest of your body, and outside factors to better understand the causes and repercussions of TMD. I invite you to look on this as a journey—both inward and outward.

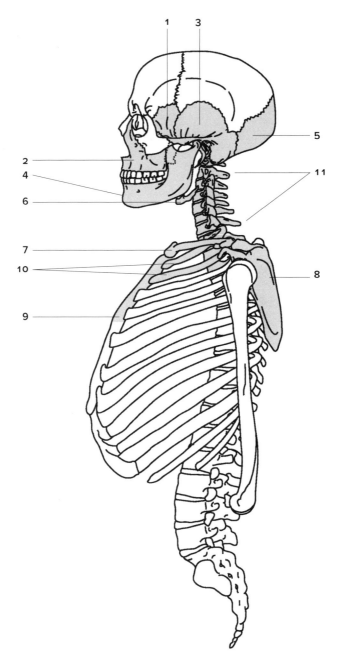

Figure 2.1: The stomatognathic system. It includes twenty-five bones:

1. Sphenoid (1)
2. Maxillae (2)
3. Temporal bones (2)
4. Mandible (1)
5. Occipital bone (1)
6. Hyoid (1)

7. Clavicles (2)
8. Scapulae (2)
9. Sternum (1)
10. Upper two ribs (right and left)
11. Top ten vertebrae (10)
    (7 cervical and upper 3 thoracic)

⚜ 2

Anatomy of Your Jaw

FROM AN EVOLUTIONARY view, the human jaw is uniquely designed to have the most possible movement and stability for a broad-spectrum omnivorous diet. Your jaw combines the strong bite of big cats (carnivores) with the lateral grinding movement of cows (herbivores) and the cutting function of rodents (using the front teeth, or incisors). When the jaw is in good alignment, there is very little pressure on the TMJs. Even with a biting force of up to 450 pounds on your molars,[1] healthy jaw dynamics enable the force to be well distributed, keeping the jaw and teeth functional and healthy.[2]

We often think of our mandible (lower jawbone) as "my jaw," as if that's all there is to it. But in fact your jaw is highly complex and intimately connected to the rest of your body. One hundred thirty-six muscles are involved in mandibular action.[3] That's sixty-eight muscle pairs above and below your mouth. Think of all of the bones those muscles attach to, and you are just beginning to get a sense of the bigger picture. The stomatognathic system—body parts necessary in biting, chewing, and swallowing—includes twenty-seven bones (figure 2.1).[4] These encompass the lower portion of your head, collarbones, shoulder blades, sternum, top two ribs on each side, and the upper half of your spine (C1–T3). When your jaw is contracted, painful, or out of alignment, the resulting limited range of motion will spread throughout your upper body and beyond over time. Let's investigate how this happens.

We will begin with a closer look at the bones immediately involved in forming your jaw, and then at the temporomandibular joints, learning more about how they function. To support our understanding of the TMJs and

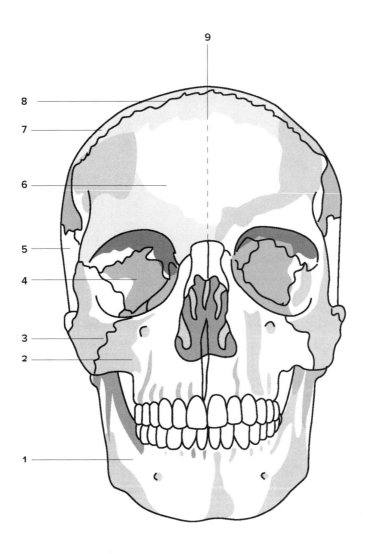

Figure 2.2a: Skull front.

1. mandible
2. maxilla
3. zygoma
4. sphenoid
5. temporal

6. frontal
7. parietal
8. coronal suture
9. sagittal suture

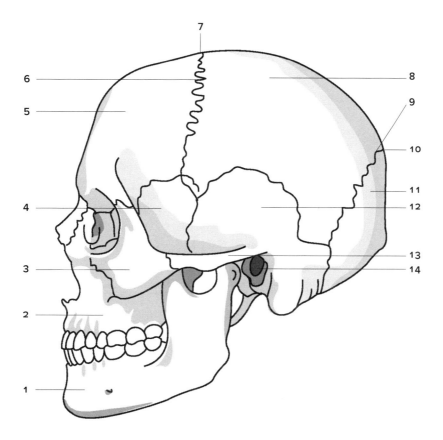

Figure 2.2b: Skull side.

1. mandible
2. maxilla
3. zygoma
4. sphenoid (greater wing)
5. frontal
6. coronal suture
7. bregma

8. parietal
9. lambdoidal suture
10. lambda
11. occiput
12. temporal
13. zygomatic arch (temporal)
14. ear canal

TMD, we'll review a few muscles of particular interest. All of the muscles included in this chapter are big players in headaches and discomfort related to TMD. Beyond anatomy and physiology, we'll explore the energetics and symbolic meanings of these parts of your body. You will gain a deepening awareness of the interconnectedness of your jaw, your mind, and the rest of your body. Perception of the integrative nature of body and mind lays a foundation for the practices presented in the yoga and mindfulness portions of this program. As you come to understand the diverse causes and repercussions of jaw tension, you will see how simple changes in your daily activities can make a big difference over time. Ultimately, you can learn to live in less pain and with greater ease through the mind-body practices presented in this book.

Wolff's Law

An important principle to keep in mind when looking at anatomy and physiology is Wolff's law. Julius Wolff, a German anatomist and surgeon, lived from 1836 to 1902.[5] He postulated that how you use your body influences how it grows and develops, particularly with regard to your skeletal structure. This is often summed up in the phrase "form follows function," meaning that the form of your bones follows how you use them. While Wolff's law is based in mathematical principles, you can see evidence of it playing out in your daily life. What happens when you stop using your body? Muscles shorten and become more rigid, and pretty quickly you have less range of motion. Since you aren't using your muscles, bone density drops, making bones more brittle and vulnerable to breaking. The changes in approach to postsurgery recovery and eldercare in the past twenty years are an expression of this principle. Bed rest used to be advocated. Now, the medical team will get you up and out of bed as quickly as possible because history has shown that lying around for days causes rapid deterioration of your body and mind. Another adage might be "Use it or lose it." As we go through the bones that make up your jaw, you will see specific examples of how the usage of your jaw—or lack thereof—can contribute to TMD.

Bones of Your Jaw
Lower Jawbone—Mandible

There is perhaps no other bone in the body that is so fundamental to our sense of self than the mandible. The jaw defines facial structure. The image of our face is what we most identify with. When we see our face in the mirror, most of us say, "Yup, that's me." The world feeds this back to us every day whether in person or through images. When you are asked to show identification, it is a picture of your face that you present. Your face is the mask you present to the world.

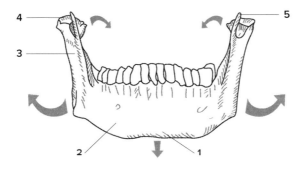

Figure 2.3: Mandible. The size and shape of the mandible (and the entire skeleton) fluctuates slightly with the cranial wave. Arrows indicate the inhalation phase of the inner tide.

1. chin   **2.** body   **3.** ramus   **4.** condyle   **5.** coronoid process

The mandible is not quite the hardest bone in your body; your thighbone holds that title. However, it is the strongest, most prominent, and most movable bone of your head. The anatomy of the mandible includes three distinct sections. The upright portion of your jaw is the *ramus* (plural: *rami*). At the top of the ramus is the *condyle* (which rests into the TMJ) and the *coronoid process* (where the temporalis muscle attaches). The two rami attach to the *body*—or horizontal portion—of the mandible. At the front center is the *chin* (also called the *mental protuberance*). In utero, the mandible starts out in two pieces, with a joint at the center of the chin that fuses over your first year. This extra pliability allows the lower jaw to adjust without breaking during birth. It also supports nursing and the resilience of a baby's head during the first year, which involves considerable growth and augmentation. Notably, humans are the only creatures with a chin.[6,7] It begs the question of why this distinctive feature would evolve. While this has yet to be resolved, the most common suggestion is that it is somehow related to mating. Have you ever been drawn to someone just because of their chin? Dimples can be surprisingly compelling.

Your mandible holds your lower teeth, forms the lower palate, supports your tongue, and is essential to taking in life-sustaining nourishment: suckling, drinking, biting, chewing, and swallowing. Numerous muscles attach to the mandible. When you use your mouth, the pushing and pulling actions of these muscles stimulate bone growth, as demonstrated by Wolff's law. Thus your jaw (and face) will fully develop in response to healthy usage. On the other hand, if we don't nurse or chew our food properly, the jaw will likely be underdeveloped.[8] Eating a diet of highly refined foods that don't require adequate chewing can lead to an overly small jaw.[9] Eventually, this can be a contributing factor to TMD and its related ailments.

Upper Jawbones—Maxillae

Your upper jaw consists of two bones, the *maxillae* (singular: *maxilla*), that are identical mirrors of one another. Together they form the roof of your mouth (upper palate), the lower portion of your eye sockets, and housing for your nose and upper teeth. The maxillae are workhorses, interacting with numerous other bones in the skull. As paired bones, they are always interacting with their twin. Additionally, each maxilla interfaces with at least eight other cranial bones—ethmoid, vomer, zygoma, palatine, interior concha, nasal, frontal, incisor. Add in the partner maxilla and you've got nine bones coming into contact with these very central bones.[10] And let's not forget the mandible, which the maxillae meet countless times throughout the day via the lower teeth. Each maxillary bone contains eight adult teeth (sixteen upper teeth total, including wisdom teeth), which are designed to work as partners to the lower teeth. Each tooth is a distinct cranial bone and, as such, is subject to absorbing tensions within its structure. The meeting of upper and lower teeth is called *occlusion*. Healthy occlusion means you are able to bite and chew your food properly. This is the first stage of digestion, and thus fundamental to your overall health and well-being. This is why healthy teeth, mouths, TMJs, and jawbones are so very important. *Malocclusion*—the poor meeting of the upper and lower teeth—plays a big role in poor health.

The continuous, multitudinous interactions the maxillae participate in make them subject to forces from a variety of directions at all times. Contrast

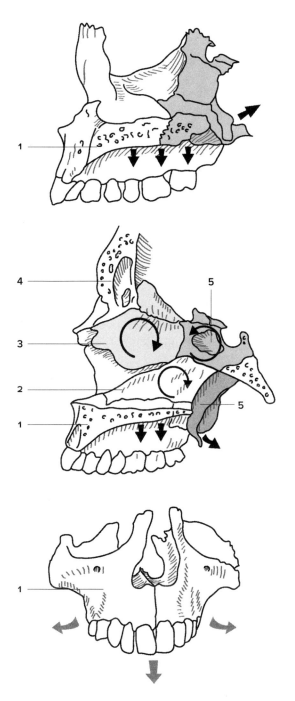

Figure 2.4: Maxillae. Arrows indicate the inhalation phase of the inner tide, impacting the roof of the mouth, sinuses, and interface with other cranial bones.

1. maxilla   **2.** vomer   **3.** ethmoid   **4.** frontal   **5.** sphenoid

this, for example, to the mandible, which connects only with the temporal bones. The result of all this contact is that the maxillae can easily become compressed, leading to discomfort in a variety of ways, as we will see.

Intriguingly, when you look at your face, you cannot immediately see the maxillae. These important bones hide behind the flashier anatomical features of our cheekbones, nasal bones, teeth, eyes, forehead, and lower jaw. Maxillae are extremely important to the facial and cranial structure. They are always there, working away, eating, talking, singing, expressing. Yet they are hardly seen or acknowledged. Somehow they seem to disappear from sight and mind—until they are distressed. Does this remind you of anyone? In addition to being infection-prone, compressed maxillae are significant contributors to migraines. (This is explored in more detail in chapter 6.) Energetically, things like not speaking your truth, biting your tongue, withholding your point of view all impact the maxillae.

The maxillae can be troublesome—they become infected more than any other cranial bone. This is largely due to the sinus cavity and teeth. The maxillae are hollow bones; the cavity inside each maxilla creates your sinuses. Clenching and grinding can cause the upper jawbones to lose their proper cranial motion (which we'll discuss in detail in the next chapter). When the maxillae lose their cranial motion, phlegm doesn't drain properly from the sinuses, which contributes to sinus infections and, potentially, root canals or tooth extraction and replacement. Your sinuses are surprisingly important. Nose breathing is far preferable to mouth breathing in many ways—it reduces the chances of infection, improves circulation of the breath, and is calming.[11] In another example of Wolff's law, excessive mouth breathing can lead to underdeveloped maxillae.[12] Imagine for a moment you grow up with allergies and your sinuses are continually blocked, causing you to breathe through your mouth much of the time, including during the night when sleeping. Innocent though this may seem, the results can include a wide range of health issues, not the least of which is sleep apnea.

Ear Bones—Temporals

The *temporals* are paired bones on either side of your head that contain the workings of your ears. The fleshy outer ears (*pinna*) sit on top of your temporal bones. The middle and inner ears are located within the bone itself. The middle ear functions as an amplifier, conducting sound into the inner ear. There,

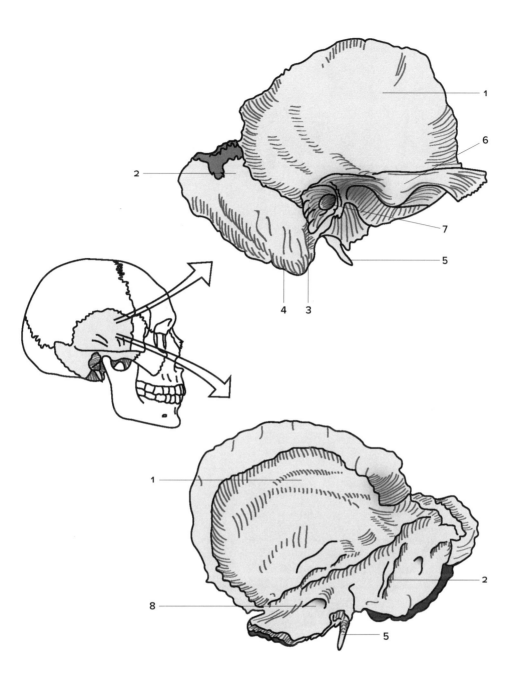

Figure 2.5: Temporal bone. This complex bone is in three pieces at birth: squamous, petrous, and tympanic. The mastoid and styloid processes develop over the first year and beyond.

1. squamous   3. tympanic   5. styloid   7. external ear canal

2. petrous   4. mastoid   6. zygomatic arch   8. internal ear canal

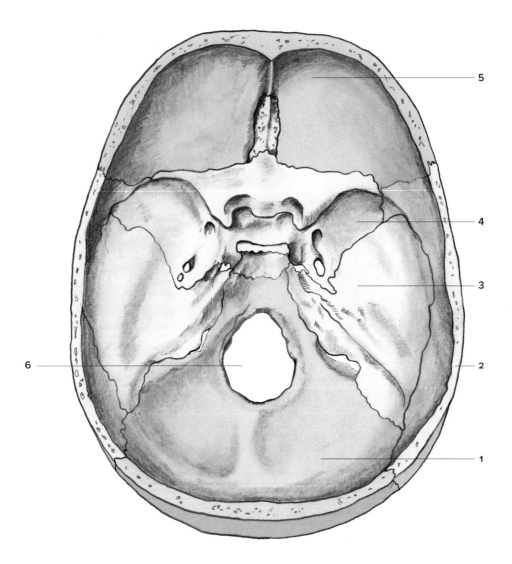

Figure 2.6: Temporal bones in cranial base. Lines represent borders between bones.
Shown here:

1. occipital bone (lower portion)
2. parietals (lower portion)
3. temporals
4. sphenoid (at center)
5. frontal bone
6. foramen magnum (opening for spine)

the *cochlea* transmute vibrational sound waves into nervous system impulses that we can interpret.[13] This is how we hear. The *vestibular labyrinth*—coupled with your upper neck—is where your sense of balance comes from.[14] You cannot easily stand, or even move, if your temporal bones and upper neck are jammed up.

The temporals are designed to work in harmony, yet their distance from one another makes them vulnerable to being thrown out of sync. As part of the cranial base, each temporal bone interfaces with five other bones: occipital, one parietal, sphenoid, one zygoma, frontal via asterion.[15] Sandwiched between these larger bones, they are subject to pressures from both the front and back of the head.

When we are born, each temporal bone is in three pieces: the petrous, tympanic, and squamous (see figure 2.5). It takes about five years for them to fuse into their adult form of a single bone. Misalignment can begin early on—from doctors' forceps, vacuum delivery, or even an apparently "perfect" natural birth with no interventions. The rotational movements of an infant preparing to emerge from the womb, combined with the pressure of contractions, can cause misalignment of the temporals relative to one another or even within the individual bone. In most cases the resilient membrane structure of a baby's head will enable natural realignment to occur within days, weeks, or months after birth. But some amount of misalignment often remains.[16] A traumatic birth overwhelms the nervous system and can lead to rigid fasciae, which often makes it harder for babies to find their natural structural balance.

Energetically, the temporals are all about equilibrium. How is your work/play balance? What is your relationship to love, contentment, suffering? Has life become all work and no joy? If temporals are out of balance, your life may well be so also. These bones will let you know they are feeling burdened and compressed through the resulting discomfort. Conditions that can impact the temporals include whiplash, slip and fall injury, a blow to the head, or chronic clenching—which is likely to happen more on one side than the other. When the temporals are thrown off, it can lead to vertigo, tinnitus, or other maladies, as we will see in the chapters that follow.

Your TMJs—Temporomandibular Joints

The temporomandibular joint (TMJ) is the largest, most prominent joint of the head—and quite possibly the most important joint of the entire body. (See figure 1.1 for a reminder of what the TMJ looks like.) Can you imagine life without it? Let's take a few minutes to consider the role the TMJs, together with your mouth, play in your life. Your jaw is put into use immediately after birth. Breastfeeding is a complex activity involving motion in the entire cranium; it activates fascial structures within your body from head to toe. (It's worth noting that bottle-feeding does not require the same complexity of effort.) Suckling provides us not only with nourishment but also connection to our mother and our world. When a baby cannot nurse, it is a life-threatening situation. Beyond survival, the oral cavity is fundamental to our sense of pleasure. Our mouths help us engage with our world in so many ways . . . through tasting, touching, smiling, kissing. We express ourselves through speech, song, and sound. Ironically, the mouth is so integral to our daily activities that we tend to take it for granted.

From an evolutionary view, the significance of the oral cavity and TMJs to your survival—as well as your ability to thrive—is reflected in how the brain has developed. Nearly half of the sensory and motor aspects of your brain are devoted to the dental area alone.[17] This means your brain is hardwired to keep close tabs on your mouth. Whatever is—or is not—happening in your mouth is continually impacting the rest of your body through brain functioning. The innervation of your jaw and face is closely associated to your feelings of safety.[18] The researcher Stephen Porges identified the *social engagement system* as our face-heart connection. Of particular importance in this are the *vagus* (cranial nerve X), which connects your heart and brain stem to the primary nerves of your face, including the *trigeminal* (cranial nerve V), which wires your jaw, *facial* (cranial nerve VII), *glossopharyngeal* (cranial nerve IX), and *accessory* (cranial nerve XI). The function of the social engagement system is to build connection to other people in order to get your needs met from a very early age, when you are not yet able to care for yourself. The primary focus is maternal bonding.

A newborn human is not self-sufficient for several years—unlike most mammals—and as a result must convey needs and build connection through expressions and sounds. Smiles and coos are purposefully endearing. The ideal situation is for baby and parents to be deeply bonded, with lots of eye contact, social engagement, coregulation, and play together. However, if parents or caregivers are unavailable in some way—through their own trauma, life experience, an unexpected accident or illness, overly busy schedules, or simply the ever-present distractions of television, computers, and phones—the baby's social nervous system may well be impacted. Instinctively, from infancy babies learn to regulate themselves in response to those around them. Their physiology will compensate for what they do not receive. Tight or imbalanced TMJs can result. In brief, *the healthy functioning of your mouth and jaw is important to, and a reflection of, the healthy functioning of your brain and nervous system.*

The intense involvement of your brain with your jaw implies a few things. When your mouth and jaw are uncomfortable and functioning poorly, the impact is often felt far beyond your face. Since your jaw is so fundamental to your well-being, when there is dysfunction or pain, the sympathetic fight-or-flight response can be activated. This reflects the body-mind's need to take action in an effort to resolve dis-

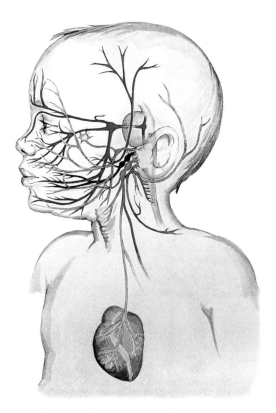

Figure 2.7: Social engagement system (SES). This system is the face-heart connection. It is formed by the linking of the vagus (cranial nerve X) with trigeminal (cranial nerve V), facial (cranial nerve VII), glossopharyngeal (cranial nerve IX), and accessory (cranial nerve XI). These cranial nerves control facial expressions and sense organs. The vagus also connects the heart, brain, and gut (internal organs).

tress. Sadly, pain and discomfort can create a self-perpetuating cycle to the point where the sympathetic nervous system forgets how to turn off and relax. We may forget what ease feels like. If this continues over time, your nervous system can be impacted in an ongoing way. For some, the relentless pain and anxiety can lead to chronic depletion of internal organs similar to post-traumatic stress disorder (PTSD). In the past twenty years the understanding of trauma and how to rewire the brain has grown considerably. The practices provided in the yoga and mindfulness sections of this book support this rewiring process.

Jaw Movements

Healthy TMJs hinge *and* glide, enabling your jaw to open, close, push forward (*protrude*), push back (*retrude*), and move sideways (*lateral motion*). The lower jaw moves forward along the saddle-shaped portion of the temporal bone. This allows for greater range of motion. Let's take a moment to test out these movements of your jaw right now. To locate your TMJs, gently place your index fingers just below your ears and at the top of your jaw. Now slide your fingers forward onto your mandible. Open and close your mouth. Do you feel your fingers being pushed outward as your mouth opens? You are on top of your TMJs. Now experiment with the movements mentioned above. You may notice one side of your jaw has more movement than the other. This is perfectly normal. Make note of these differences. They will become useful information as we continue the journey of unraveling jaw tension. We will explore them closely when we get into in the Mapping Your Body exercise on page 115 and the rest of part two.

When the TMJs are properly aligned, they should be stress-free, with virtually no pressure on the joints when chewing.[19] The pressure drops through the teeth into the (very strong) jawbone. Similar to knees, hips, and ankles, when things are lined up and moving properly, the joints don't take the stress. It's when things are not aligned that problems arise.

Muscles of Interest

The four primary muscles of mastication are the *masseter, temporalis*, and *lateral and medial pterygoids*. There are two of each of these muscles—one each on the right and left sides of your face—and they all attach to the ramus portion of your lower jaw. Since these are muscles for biting and chewing, they are all in some way involved in closing your mouth, except for the lateral pterygoid, which opens your mouth along with the hyoid muscles. All of these can be factors in headaches, both directly and indirectly through trigger points. As a result, it's helpful to know where they are and how to release them. These muscles are a special focus of the facial self-massage sequence offered at the end of part one. The descriptions here will inform your daily experience of your face, mouth, and jaw.

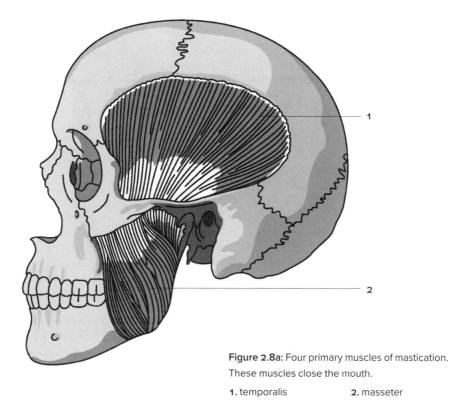

Figure 2.8a: Four primary muscles of mastication. These muscles close the mouth.

1. temporalis   **2.** masseter

Masseter

The strongest muscle in your body is the *masseter* (figure 2.8a). Its main job is to close your mouth, giving your bite a lot of power. When only one side is activated, the masseter contributes to the sideways motion necessary for grinding up whole grains. If you look at herbivores like cows or horses, this muscle will be very developed. In humans, an overdeveloped masseter can contribute to clenched jaws, broken teeth, a tight neck, and painful, damaged TMJs. The masseter begins at the lower edge of your cheekbone or zygomatic arch—which includes portions of the maxillae, zygomata, and temporal bones. It ends at the lower angle of your mandible, covering the upright portion of your lower jawbone. The masseter is a dense, bunchy, fibrous muscle. It often likes deep, steady pressure massage to help it relax.

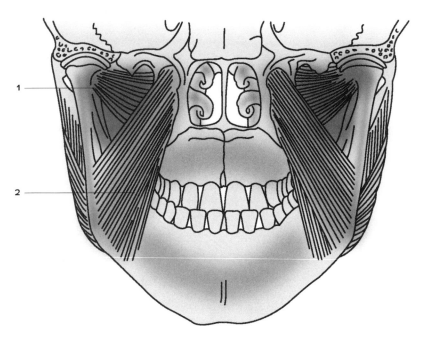

Figure 2.8b: Four primary muscles of mastication. The lateral pterygoid opens the mouth.

1. lateral pterygoid   **2.** medial pterygoid

Temporalis

Your largest chewing muscle is the *temporalis* (figure 2.8a). It is so large that it overlaps with several bones—including the temporal, parietal, frontal, sphenoid, and mandible—which means it can be a big factor in headaches, particularly those on the side of your head (figure 2.2b). Imagine a wide, stretchy rubber strap pulled tightly over several puzzle pieces . . . and then tighten the strap even more. What happens to the pieces of the puzzle? They get all bunched up and jumbled together so that they can no longer lie flat side by side. This is like the bones of your head, being compressed by a very tight and overworked temporalis muscle that just doesn't know how to let go.

The temporalis has a beautiful fan shape and is located on either side of your head. Like the masseter, the temporalis helps close your mouth. Additionally it pulls your lower jaw back (retrusion) as you chew. The temporalis begins at a bony ridge called the *temporal fossa*, midway along the parietal bones that form the top of your head. It ends on the upper portion of your mandible, just below your cheekbones, in front of the TMJ at the coronoid process of your mandible. Curiously, this is just below where the masseter begins, so these two powerful muscles overlap slightly, a design which contributes to the strong clamping-down bite of your jaw (think tigers). This muscle is very well developed in carnivores. In humans, the fibers of the temporalis run in three different directions—vertical, slanting, and horizontal—allowing it to both lift and retract your mandible. Distinct from the masseter, the temporalis is a flat, shallow muscle that prefers lighter pressures and can be sensitive to touch.

Medial Pterygoid

The next two chewing muscles—the *medial and lateral pterygoid*—are internal, and thus are not easily accessed from the outside of your head and face. It's helpful to know where they are, though, because they respond to energetic contact and clear intention and can still be released. The *medial pterygoid* is located behind the back of your mouth (figure 2.8b). It begins at the inner surface of the lateral pterygoid plate, which is the lower portion of the sphenoid bone. It ends on the inner surface of the mandible, under your lower palate. This muscle's job is to close your mouth, push your lower jaw forward (protrusion), and move it sideways (lateral excursion)—three actions that are integral to chewing.

Lateral Pterygoid

Have you ever woken up and been unable to open your mouth? It's very likely your *lateral pterygoid* was in spasm (figure 2.8b). This muscle is essential to your mouth's ability to open. It attaches directly into the TMJ—which means it has more impact on how well the joint is working than any other muscle. It also assists its friend the medial pterygoid with the forward and sideways movement of your lower jaw. The lateral pterygoid muscle has two portions. It begins at both the greater wing and the outer surface of the lateral pterygoid of sphenoid bone (the bone behind your eyes) and ends at the disc of the TMJ and on the condyle of the mandible, which rests in the TMJ.

Let's take a closer look at this very special little muscle. Less than an inch long, an upset lateral pterygoid makes itself known in a variety of ways. Since its upper portion attaches to the disc of the TMJ, if it's overly tight, it can actually pull the disc out of the joint, making it difficult and painful to open your mouth. The lower portion of the muscle inserts on the condyle of the mandible, which rests in the TMJ—so once again a contracted lateral ptery-goid can make it hard to use this joint, even contributing to dislocation.

Since the lateral pterygoid begins at your sphenoid bone, it is associated with vision and visual disturbances. We literally see through the sphenoid—it is the bone that holds your eyes. When this muscle is out of balance, it can distort vision—both the outer and inner varieties. Dyslexia is one possible result. Looking through a symbolic lens, we can tune in to the energetics of what a tight lateral pterygoid might be expressing. For example, what is the gap between what you see and what you say? Do you trust your vision? Do you speak your truth? Or has your need to please others and feel safe resulted in biting your tongue, swallowing your words, and clenching your jaw? What is your relationship to your visionary self, your aspirations and goals for this lifetime? Have you forgotten your dreams, hiding them away in Pandora's box, tossing away the key? Your heart may be speaking to you through lat-eral pterygoid, whispering in your ear, *Speak up! How you feel matters! Let your heart be known . . . Now is the time!* I am reminded of the Rumi poem,

> The breezes at dawn have secrets to tell you
> Don't go back to sleep!
> You must ask for what you really want.
> Don't go back to sleep!
> People are going back and forth
> across the doorsill where the two worlds touch,
> The door is round and open
> Don't go back to sleep![20]

Lateral pterygoid is also a factor in scoliosis. The sphenoid bone is at the very center of the head, directly above the spine. When it is out of balance, partic-ularly at a young age, it can influence how the spine grows and develops. A torqued sphenoid lays a foundation for a torqued spine.[21]

Widening the lens beyond the mouth and head, the lateral pterygoid often mirrors contraction in the pelvic floor muscles—piriformis, coccygeus, and particularly psoas. These muscles are energetically connected: Relaxing the lateral pterygoid muscle can release the psoas and pelvic floor. In fact, one of the most effective ways to relieve chronic acute sciatica is through an intraoral release of the lateral pterygoid muscle. Similarly, releasing the pel-vic floor can release lateral pterygoid. It may happen that when you release

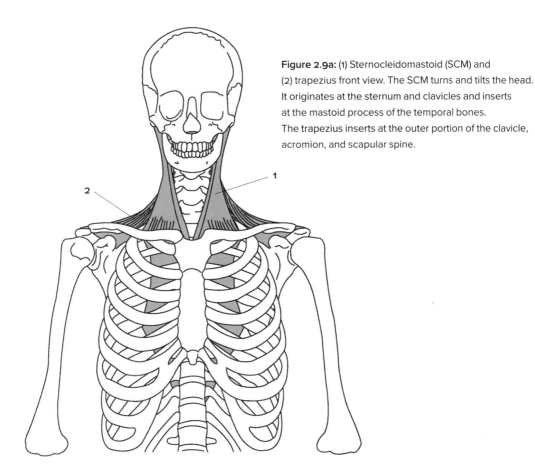

Figure 2.9a: (1) Sternocleidomastoid (SCM) and (2) trapezius front view. The SCM turns and tilts the head. It originates at the sternum and clavicles and inserts at the mastoid process of the temporal bones. The trapezius inserts at the outer portion of the clavicle, acromion, and scapular spine.

this muscle, you begin to cry. This is due to its unusual psycho-emotional quality. It has a special connection with our sense of safety and vulnerability. This reciprocal connection between the hips and jaw is explored more in subsequent chapters. It also informs our yoga practice in part two.

Other Significant Muscles— Sternocleidomastoid and Trapezius

Now let's check out a few muscles that connect your jaw and head with your neck, chest, and back. The *sternocleidomastoid*'s name tells you just where this muscle resides. It originates at your sternum and collarbones and inserts at the mastoid process of your temporal bone (see figure 2.9a). To feel this muscle we'll begin at the end. Gently place your index fingers below your ears and at the top of your jaw. Now move your fingers backward to feel the firm

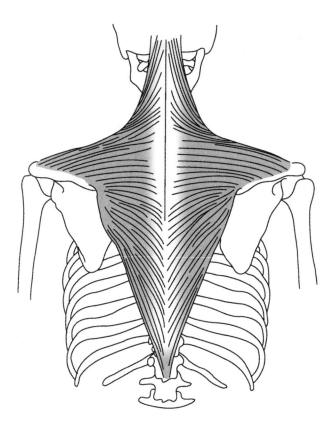

Figure 2.9b: Trapezius back view. The trapezius originates at the occiput and all thoracic vertebrae (1–12). It attaches to cervical vertebrae via the nuchal ligament. It inserts on the clavicles, acromion, and spine of the scapulae.

bone just behind and below your ears. This is your mastoid process where the SCM ends. Slide your fingers down to the lowest point of the bone, and then onto your neck. These are your SCMs. Let your fingers follow this pathway down the sides of your neck to your collarbones and sternum, where the SCM begins (figure 2.9a).

The SCM allows you to lift and turn your head. Since the SCM attaches to your temporal bone, it can become very tight from clenching. When this happens, you'll find it difficult—and maybe painful—to perform the simple and essential task of turning your head. The SCM is also involved with lifting your sternum, helping with inhalation. You must stabilize your shoulders for this to happen (and you'll practice doing this in the yoga exercises in part two). If your neck and shoulders are chronically contracted, the SCM will be overly tight, which contributes to restricted breathing.

At the back of your head and upper back you'll find your *trapezius* muscles (plural: *trapezii*) (see figure 2.9b). The name comes from the beautiful trapezoid resulting from two large triangular muscles that spread outward from the spine and cover your upper back and neck. A friend can help you find this muscle by placing their hands at the back of your head, gently sweeping their hands down your neck and across the top of your shoulders to the outer edges of the collarbones, and then moving across your shoulder blades and upper back. Following the diamond shape of the trapezius, their hands will meet two-thirds of the way down your spine. The trapezius is affected by conditions that impact the neck, including jaw tension, whiplash, etc. When we clench, we tend to find ourselves unconsciously jutting the jaw forward and extending the neck. This is a part of a defensive, aggressive posture: tightened fists, raised shoulders, contracted muscles ready to fight. Even if we don't actually come to blows, the patterning to defend ourselves and our pack resides deep within our being. Overdeveloped traps result in having your shoulders scrunched up around your ears. Somehow your neck seems to have disappeared. It's hiding under traps that just don't know how to let go.

The trapezii allow you to shrug your shoulders up and down, throw a ball, broaden your back, and extend your neck—or at least they do so when the shoulders are stabilized, as we'll explore in the core actions in chapter 10. When your traps are tight, your neck and upper back will likely be achy. Your shoulders will feel stiff and be hard to move. And you may develop headaches that start at the back of your head, sometimes wrapping up and over the top. It's worth noting that your SCM and traps share a common attachment point. They both connect to your clavicles. This means that occasionally, they share muscle fibers. Even though one is at the front of your body and the other at your back, they can become intertwined. In the case of chronic tension, one can get the other going—not unlike when one of your kids is upset and agitated and then somehow manages to recruit their sibling into their drama. This can make for a lot of misery in your body—headaches at the side and back of your head simultaneously.

A superficial muscle, each trapezius begins on the occipital bone at the base of your skull and extends along the upper two-thirds of your spine, attaching to your vertebrae all the way down to thoracic 12. This elegant muscle is so large, it has three distinct sections. The upper portion raises and upwardly rotates your shoulder blades—important for raising your arms overhead and throwing overhand. It also lengthens your neck when your shoulders are stabilized. This part of the trapezius extends from the base of your skull and the vertebrae of your neck (via the nuchal ligament) and wraps over the top of your shoulders—actually, we could say it *forms* your shoulder top. It ends at the outer edge of your collarbones. The muscle fibers in this section run downward, spreading across your upper back like a fan.

The middle section covers your upper back, extending from cervical 7 through thoracic 3. It expands outward from the spine across your ribs and shoulder blades, ending at the upper portion of your scapulae (acromion and superior crest). These muscle fibers mostly run horizontally across the upper back, allowing you to pull your shoulder blades together. The lower portion acts as an antagonist to the upper part, opposing it through lowering your shoulder blades. It also supports the upper portion with upward rotation. This section originates at your middle back (thoracic 4–12) and inserts at the upper part of the shoulder blades. These muscle fibers orient up and out, a lower fan meeting the upper fan.

Poor posture is a big factor in trapezius overuse, resulting in chronic tension. When you sit at the computer, is your back rounded, with your head pushed forward and your chest drooping? If you have poor vision, it will likely cause you to do this even more. Now imagine yourself unconsciously clenching your way through your workday . . . You'll have some very contracted muscles ready to complain. I hate to say it, but slouching is not your friend when it comes to trapezius muscles. In part two, we will explore ways to undo this stress posture.

We'll be referring back to your jaw's anatomy and physiology as we delve more deeply into the causes and repercussions of TMD. As you continue learning, perhaps you'll begin to notice your body in a new way, feeling a bit more intimate with the different parts that make up the whole. Maybe you'll begin to view your aches and pains in a new light. Your body and mind are working hard to support you in your life, day in, day out. Can you turn toward your experience with curiosity and inquisitiveness? Just how is it that all of these pieces come together . . . to form *you*?

3

The Inner Tide and Cranial Wave

IN THIS CHAPTER we will explore a few fundamental concepts of craniosacral bodywork and note some parallels between craniosacral, yoga, and mindfulness. These concepts will further your understanding of how jaw tension can have a wide range of impacts throughout your body. Something each of these disciplines share is that they are based in experiential understanding. While terminology has developed specific to each, they all begin with the direct experience of body and mind. They just describe it differently. It's helpful to recognize these disciplines developed in different areas around the globe and express unique ways of thinking about the fascinating experience of being human and alive. Another way to think about the intersection of these three practices is to consider this: The human heart was beating before anyone found a pulse, recorded its rate, and gave it a name. In fact, your heartbeat continues to be described by multifarious names in cultures around the world. Every society has its own expression of what the heart is and what it does—yet we are all talking about the same thing.

These traditions encourage us to trust our intuition. Mindfulness, yoga, and craniosacral each support a deepening of present-moment awareness. When we are rooted in direct experience, moment by moment, we gain a depth of confidence. This confidence supports intuitive understanding. Learning to trust our intuition is essential to recognizing what we know to be true—and honoring what we don't know. Studying is important, and terminology serves a purpose in helping us to articulate our experience. But ultimately these systems share the view that intuition is the deepest form of knowing.

Additionally, each of these modalities recognizes the healing nature of accessing a transcendent state of mind. Transcendence—or big mind—is equated with unconditional love and release from our deep need for belonging. When we abide in big mind, we feel connected with everyone and everything. Our sense of smallness and separation fall away. These traditions all appreciate that transcendence is available within our mundane experience at all times. Your cells are continually responding to every experience, moment by moment by moment. Craniosacral, yoga, and mindfulness facilitate the integration of life experience, leading to harmony of mind and body for greater ease, contentment, and overall well-being. These practices offer a pathway toward abiding in a state of *agape*—universal love and intimacy with all things.

Gaia: Self-Regulation and the Tide

The ancient Greeks understood the earth to be a self-regulating organism: a goddess called Gaia. Looking through this metaphoric lens, we can see that oceans, lakes, ponds, rivers, and streams form the fluid body of our earth. The moon's gravitational pull draws ocean water from one side of the earth to the other. This tidal force is expressed twice a day—as high and low tides—and fluctuates with the seasons, influenced by the relative distance between earth and moon.

The oceanic tide provides circulation of Gaia's fluid body, washing and cleansing her shores, spreading nutriment through her seas, and furnishing a fundamental rhythm that supports the cycle of life. All levels of life benefit from this circulation, from the minute to the massive. Kelp forests, coral, crabs, fish, and even whales depend on the tide for food, nourishment, and regulation. The timing of sea creatures' procreation is synchronized with the tide.

But the tide doesn't end at the seashore. As we move further from the coastline, the impact of the tide can still be seen. At first glance lakes and rivers may not appear to have a tide, but they do fluctuate with the moon cycle, albeit on a smaller scale. Salmon migration is a beautiful example of how the tide extends deeply onto the land-based areas of Gaia. Born in a stream as much as two hundred miles from the ocean, they swim thousands of miles in their lifetime until, years later, they are pulled by the moon to return to the very same stream where their life began. The tide influences weather patterns, contributing to cycles of wind and rain that move across the continents and around the earth. Looking closely we can see the tide's effects across the entire planet.

All living beings are integral aspects of Gaia—including you and me. As such, we contain within us a microcosmic expression of the macrocosm of our Mother Earth. Our fluid bodies consist of veins and arteries that function as rivers and streams. Examples of ponds and lakes include our intestines, bladder, and heart. Our sophisticated membrane structure, formed by connective tissue or *fascia*, allows for head to toe connection, maintaining the fluid, oceanic quality within. Craniosacral understands the fluid body to be more than the sum of its parts. It is inherently intelligent and supportive. It serves as an organizing principle, containing a life force or *potency*—the equivalent of *prana* in yoga or *chi* in Chinese medicine. The fluid body provides protection to the organism as a whole and holds healing intentions for your being.

Similar to the earth's tide, there is a tide within your body. The *inner tide*, or *cranial wave*, is essentially a circulatory system that keeps all levels of your structure supple, pliable, nourished, and fully alive. This force is constantly working to wash away blockages within your body on every level. The inner tide's subtle, constant motion has both wavelike and tidal qualities of rhythmic pulsation and regulatory circulation that pass through every bodily structure from head to toe: bones, internal organs, fluids, membranes, and connective tissue. It affects all aspects of body and mind—our physical, emotional, psychological, and energetic state of being. When this circulatory system is obstructed or interfered with, disharmony results.

The inner tide is not dependent on or influenced by the external movements of your body. It ebbs and flows whether you are sleeping or awake, standing, walking, bending, doing yoga poses, going for a run, meditating, or sitting in a meeting. Much of the time—although not always—its movement is coordinated with your breathing. Inhalation is an expansion phase and exhalation a releasing phase. One way to envision the inner tide is to think of a hologram. As you breathe in, imagine your body subtly broadening side to side, narrowing front to back, and becoming just a tiny bit shorter as your connection to earth grows. As you breathe out, envision your body subtly narrowing side to side, broadening front to back, and growing just a tiny bit taller as your connection to the sky expands. In your limbs the tide is expressed as a subtle rotation. Your arms and legs gently rotate externally

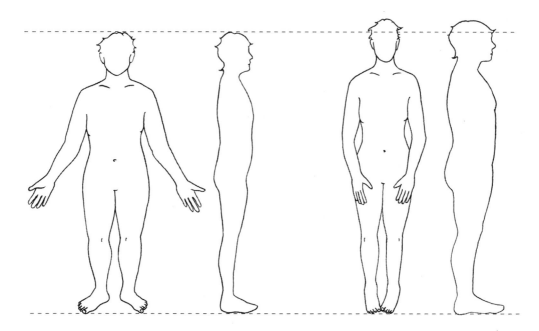

Figure 3.1: The tidal body.
The entire body fluctuates with tidal movement. With inhalation/flexion/external rotation, the body broadens side to side, narrows front to back, and shortens top to bottom. Limbs externally rotate. With exhalation/extension/internal rotation, the body narrows side to side, broadens front to back, and lengthens top to bottom. The limbs internally rotate.

during inhalation (expansion phase) and internally during exhalation (releasing phase). The rotational quality is transmitted through all the tissues but felt most strongly at the skeletal level. Understanding and working with the inner tide can help you find greater harmony in your being, including relief from jaw tension. The tide is too subtle to be seen with normal vision, but you can learn to experience it through practices like yoga and mindfulness. This is explored in detail in the core action of the hips (page 133).

Tidal Frequency

The inner tide functions at three distinct rates that correspond to states of mind. The fastest rate is called the *Cranial Rhythmic Impulse (CRI), cranial pulse, Traube-Hering wave,* or *cranial wave.* The cranial wave pulses through your body eight to fourteen times a minute in normal waking consciousness.[1] A single wave lasts about six seconds, with three seconds of expansion (inhale), followed by three seconds of release (exhale). Compared to a typical heart rate—about sixty beats a minute—the cranial wave is quiet and slow. It's also extremely subtle: The amplitude of this movement is only forty microns. To give a relative perspective, a sheet of paper is about one hundred microns thick.

As we relax, the tide slows. *Mid-tide*, or *fluid tide*, occurs 2.5 times per minute, which is a twenty-four-second cycle: twelve seconds of expanding (inhale), and twelve seconds of releasing (exhale).[2] In mid-tide we feel connected to others and our environment, which means we feel less separate or isolated. Emotions are simpler, arising and passing in a way that is natural and uncontrolled, fluid.

As we keep relaxing, the tide can slow to a cycle of one hundred seconds— fifty seconds of expansion (inhale), and fifty seconds of releasing (exhale). This is called *long tide*, a state of tranquility.[3] In this state, we feel intimate with all things. The truth that we are a part of everything is keenly apparent. A term coined by the Vietnamese Buddhist monk Thich Nhat Hanh—*interbeing*—captures the essence of this quality. We may experience it in meditation, when we are in nature, or when we are simply at ease. There is no misery in long tide: only peace, contentment, and joyful connection. It is available to all of us at any time. Practices like mindfulness and yoga can help cultivate the inner calm that enables long tide to be expressed more frequently.

The inner tide gives us a profound, well-researched demonstration of how our physiology and consciousness are interdependent. Despite the increasing subtlety of the cranial wave, mid-tide, and long tide, you can experience them within your own body. One of the ways you can recognize them is by simply noticing your state of mind, as described above. If you are at ease, you are in mid-tide. If you are tranquil, feeling connected and a part of everything, you are in long tide. If you are distraught, ill at ease, agitated, or disconnected, you are in CRI.

You have probably experienced all of these states many times in your life. Have you ever noticed that you relax more easily by the seashore? The rhythmic pulsation of the waves breaking against the shore informs your being, the external tide informing your inner tide. Reconnecting with nature, we lose our separateness. This is a reflection of the inner tidal experience manifesting. Craniosacral gives us the language and understanding to quantify the ways that our environment, experiences, and the people we surround ourselves with impact our physiology.

Another idea fundamental to craniosacral is the recognition that the living human skull is not fused but rather pliable and highly responsive to pressures from both inside and outside the body. The joints between the cranial bones—or sutures—gap very slightly in response to the movement of the inner tide or cranial wave. The alignment of the cranial bones can be supported and adjusted by skillful touch. This is an important basis of cranial work. The quality of touch that is most often used is exceedingly light, approximately five grams or the weight of a nickel.

Origins of Craniosacral

The osteopath Dr. William Sutherland, who graduated in 1900 from the American School of Osteopathy in Kirksville, Missouri, is largely considered to be the grandfather of craniosacral work. He grew curious about the resilient nature of the cranium through a moment of intuition in his final year as a medical student. Looking at a disarticulated skull on display, the thought occurred to him that the edges of the temporal bones seemed to indicate movement—they were "beveled, like the gills of a fish."[4] The notion was a bit unsettling as it was not encompassed by his education . . . and yet, in the way that intuition sometimes has with us, he couldn't forget it. So he turned toward the thought and began to explore how he might either prove—or disprove—this possibility. A curious and meticulous scientist, Sutherland experimented first on his own body to refine his hypotheses and then used these experiences to develop techniques to help others. His work between 1900 and 1950, along with that of other osteopaths, formed the basis of cranial osteopathy in North America.

His was a living laboratory. While conducting research on himself, Sutherland used a 1900s American football helmet made of padded leather and modified it to apply pressure on individual cranial bones. He then mindfully noted his physiological and psycho-emotional responses. To better understand the relationship of the pelvis and sacrum to the cranium, Sutherland created a device using a baseball mitt with ropes and pulleys to create traction on his sacrum.[5] He experienced distinct responses to these experiments, which confirmed the pliable, resilient quality of the living skull as well as a clear connection to the pelvis. The impact of the experiments not only affected Dr. Sutherland's physical structure but also his quality of mind. More than once he found he couldn't think straight, and he even felt he'd "gone a little wacky."[6] Thankfully, he was able to undo the disturbances he created within himself. Admittedly he did enlist the help of his wife, Adah, more than once to assist him in getting himself fully back together. When he needed an extra hand for his experiments, she was called in to help him out . . . and to uncrank the pressure if he should become unable to do so.[7] His work has since been validated and replicated many times in more modern settings,[8] and it was integral to the development of craniosacral technique.

The Brain Breath—Building a Bridge to Yoga

In 1996 I walked into a yoga class at the Iyengar Yoga Institute in San Francisco. Ramanand Patel was the teacher. I had just recently moved to San Francisco after three years of living in spiritual communities and Buddhist monasteries, doing a lot of meditation and yoga practice. My mind and body had transformed very rapidly during those years. Previously unrecognized trauma had teased itself to the surface and was primed for release—only I didn't quite know that yet. What I did know was I had some chronic tension patterns. In this classroom, I was about to experience a deeply transformative modality that had a profound impact on my life.

The Iyengar system of yoga is unique with regard to its use of props. And the San Francisco Institute was a fully equipped studio. Before I knew it, we were using multiple blankets, blocks, straps, chairs, and benches with such precision it felt like surgery without the knife. I had never experienced anything like this.

On my second or third class, while I was hanging upside down on a sling, my lower back went into spasm, and I couldn't get myself out of the pose. I quietly asked for help as the teacher walked by. Somehow Ramanand saw what was happening in my body. After helping me to get down from my perch, he guided an assistant to put me in a series of supported postures. And then, out of nowhere, I began to cry. Crying became sobbing, and sobbing became wailing. A dam had broken within me, resulting in breath flooding into parts of my body that had been previously off-limits to my own mind. I remain tremendously grateful for this experience of becoming reacquainted with my body. Something that had been inaccessible to me was now available for a deeper healing. I continued to work with Ramanand over the next decade, both privately and in public classes.

During this time I also enrolled in the Visionary Craniosacral Work program led by Hugh Milne. I was delighted and inspired by his frequent reference to yogic and Buddhist philosophy and practices in both his textbook and his trainings. Additionally, the visionary training was a wonderful support for cultivating greater trust in my intuition. Hugh's approach inspired me to draw connections between the disciplines of craniosacral, yoga, and mindfulness, each of which has been an integral part of my life ever since. Similar to my experience with Ramanand, Hugh seemed to have a grasp of physiology that was something different than I had come across. My work with these two teachers was complemented by my meditation teachers, Ruth Denison and Ajahn Pasanno. Ruth had a very special way of guiding us deep within our being. And Ajahn Pasanno never failed to keep me grounded in both the mundane and the transcendent. Receiving guidance from these four individuals over many years has contributed to an exquisite experience of living physiology.

As I learned about the origins of craniosacral and Dr. Sutherland's experiments, I couldn't help but notice similarities to the application of props in the Iyengar system. For example, the use of a head wrap was common in Ramanand's classes. This is an Indian-style ACE bandage—which has less elastic than the American version, making it a gentle support—wrapped carefully around your head. It can be used with precision by inserting a twist here, a knot there . . . A seed or other small object, specifically placed, can release restrictions between cranial bones, membranes, or other levels of tissues in the head. This can be beneficial for relieving headaches and sinus blockage or infection, as well as structural imbalances in your head and neck. It is relaxing and supports calming of the sense organs—eyes, ears, nose, and throat in particular—facilitating a calm state of being.

One day when I was working with Ramanand, he pointed out that my tailbone was stuck. Who knew?! To release this we removed a yoga wall rope and looped it around my hips, pulling the triple fisherman's knot through the rope to secure it. I then lay down on the floor on my back. The knot landed against the tailbone—which felt terrific, by the way. A yoga strap was then run through the loose end of the yoga rope just below the knot and subsequently passed through an eye screw bolted into the wall near the floor. I bent my knees slightly as we tightened the yoga strap just enough . . . so that when I straightened my legs, the hip bones were stabilized and slightly compressed at the front, freeing the sacrum at the back. A delightful traction was created on my sacrum, freeing my tailbone. What a relief! Having never known a free tailbone until that moment, I would not have realized it needed releasing. But I got that *something* was off. Such is the quest for healing. We may not fully know what we need or where we are going, but there is the longing, the desire for wellness, the intuition that things could be different or better, and the inspiration to seek relief.

My experience with the yoga rope and strap reminded me of Dr. Sutherland's baseball-mitt traction. I asked Ramanand about his training and whether it included techniques developed by Dr. Sutherland. He told me he had never experienced or studied craniosacral, though he had heard of it. His work with yoga props was based on his training directly with BKS Iyengar, his understanding of Ayurveda, and his curiosity and interest in materials from his early career as a civil engineer.

The Winds of Life

Ramanand frequently mentioned "brain breath" and the *vayus* ("winds" or life force energy) in his classes. He explained the rhythmic oscillation of the brain within the head very clearly. His description was strikingly similar to what I experienced in my cranial training. The difference was he was describing it from inside his body. He didn't reference cranial anatomy or what someone else touching a body from the outside might notice. He would guide us in the experience of the subtle oscillation of the brain hemispheres for several minutes while we were in supported poses. "On the in-breath, the hemispheres of the brain release toward one another. On the out-breath, the hemispheres of the brain release away from one another, toward the circumference of the skull."

Iyengar Yoga recognizes the brain breath to be an expression of the *vayus*. *Vayus* literally translates as "winds"—they are an explanation of the movement of life force energy, or prana, which is a cornerstone concept in Ayurveda.[9] The brain breath, or prana vayu, is one of five breaths or winds governing energy flow within the body. Ramanand would describe the movement of the other vayus at various times during class, in particular during our Savasana pose at the end. Once again, the experience resonated with my craniosacral training. He described a subtle pervasive movement downward on the inhale and upward on the exhale. He also explained the relationship between the *apana* (pelvic breath), *udana* (thoracic breath), and prana (brain breath) vayus with regard to movement of energy within the body. He recognized that clearing the pelvic breath (apana vayu, which governs elimination and downward movement from hips to feet) would in turn clear the thoracic

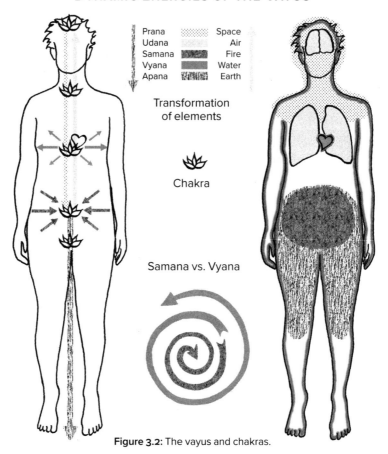

Figure 3.2: The vayus and chakras.

breath (udana vayu—governing upward movement from hips to shoulders), which in turn would release the brain breath (prana vayu, which governs downward movement from head to hips). This deepened my understanding of why opening the hips and subtly rotating the heads of the thighbones in the hip sockets could have a series of benefits that manifested far from the hips—including freeing the lungs, clearing the sinuses, and resolving headaches. Beyond theory, I witnessed the impact on my classmates, experienced the benefits directly in my body, and was able to replicate this in my work with students. I now had another explanation for why a client's sinuses cleared when I released their sacrum! In craniosacral this is explained via the *core link*, which we'll go into in chapters 5 and 7.

The final two vayus are *vyana* and *samana*. Vyana vayu governs circulation, movement from the heart (or center) to the periphery. Samana vayu governs absorption, movement from the periphery (skin and environment) to the center. These two balance and oppose one another, in the same way that udana vayu balances and opposes the combination of apana and prana vayus. Together, these five winds form a subtle body movement similar to a hologram. The body expands and contracts, broadens and narrows, shortens and lengthens . . . rhythmically, independent of gross body movement, whether sleeping or awake. The vayus were first written about by the ancient rishis in the Vedas and Upanishads. These texts lay a foundation for the healing science of Ayurveda. As a cranial practitioner and also a yoga student, I am fascinated by the similarities between these systems. Could they possibly be the same thing? While the language used to represent them is different, the felt experience is where the similarities lie.

Cranial Sutures and Brain Breath

Since it bears repeating, I will reemphasize that cranial concepts were—and continue to be—developed in response to direct perception that is rooted in the clinical experience of the practitioner. It is not the other way around. Cranial concepts describe natural phenomena that occur in every living being, regardless of gender, ethnicity, place of birth, or even species.

Returning to Dr. Sutherland's experiments, we have learned that your head and your brain, along with the rest of the body, change shape continually. The bones of your head are intimately intertwined with one another through their cranial movement patterns. The tide allows the *sutures* (places where bones of your head meet) to gently and repeatedly gap, expand, and release. Your head, brain, and whole body slightly broaden and flatten, becoming shorter and wider in the expansion phase (inhalation) (see figure 3.3.). Then they each slightly elongate and narrow, together with the whole body becoming taller during the releasing phase (exhalation) (see figure

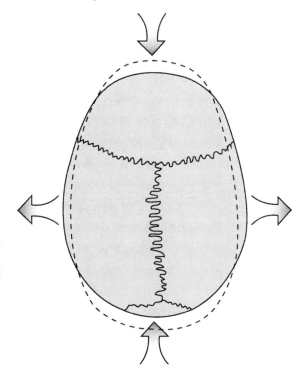

Figure 3.3: Tidal fluctuation of the skull. Arrows indicate inhalation.

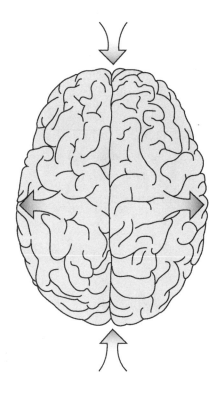

3.4). This means the bones themselves actually expand and release, changing size and shape on the order of forty microns several times a minute. In addition, each individual cranial bone has a distinct movement pattern in harmony with the movement of the entire skull.

Some of the skull's sutures are *interdigitated*, meaning the bones interrelate with a zipper-like joint as pictured in figure 3.3. It is fascinating to note that, like fingerprints, the pattern of interdigitation is unique to each person. The skull of a newborn has no interdigitated sutures. These will develop over the course of a lifetime. Thus, sutures are a record of your unique experience and history—a road map to your life.

Figure 3.4: Tidal fluctuations of the brain. Arrows indicate inhalation.

Applying the Inner Tide to Jaw Tension

There are a number of ways that understanding the inner tide can help our work with jaw tension. As mentioned above, the tide is constantly passing through the entire body. While your body may appear solid, on a subtler level it is constantly fluctuating, expanding, and contracting with the tide. A restriction in one part of your body can be transmitted to a seemingly distant area through the fluid body, in the same way that radioactive water released from Fukushima in Japan can show up in fish in Seattle. Or that whales who summer in the arctic waters of Alaska spend the winter off Baja, six thousand miles away. Imagine a single drop of water falling on a pond. That single drop sends ripples out across the entire pond, eventually reaching every shore. This is like the tide traveling through your fluid body. Nothing remains untouched.

The cranial wave reveals how interconnected the entire body is and shows us how a tight jaw can influence your head, shoulders, hips, or even your feet. If one or more bones have limited movement due to chronic tension patterns—as in the case of TMD—this will impinge on other bones, which will in turn affect fluids, membranes, and organs. Here is another analogy:

Imagine you are holding a water balloon. If you pinch two sides of the water balloon, what happens? It will be forced to change shape. The fluid inside of the balloon has been influenced by the force your hand is applying to the outside of the balloon. In a similar way, if the TMJs are chronically tight, this will impact the cranial bones, affecting your facial structure, membranes, and the fluid balance of the head. Our bodies are 50–65 percent water, and our brains are 73 percent water. Fluid dynamics play an important role in our physiology. Even brain functioning can be disturbed by chronic jaw tension. Tight muscles pulling on cranial bones can tug on the membranes inside your head, which hold your brain. When those membranes are pulled tightly, this impacts how your brain works. We might liken the experience to wearing a suit that's too tight. How do *you* function in clothes you cannot move freely in? Your brain cares about its environment and does not perform well when things are off.

The capacity to work with the tide and the gapping of the sutures is a distinctive aspect of cranial work. When we encourage the sutures to gently open, this is an invitation to reset the cranium—and in the process, to release life experience, shifting our relationship to what has been and what is yet to come. Suture release cannot be forced but rather arises through careful awareness and receptivity. It is a profound moment. Long-held trauma may be discharged. Babies often cry briefly as sutures gap, perhaps in response to feeling a change in their being. And then deep calm arises—quiet, stillness, ease.

The tide shows us how jaw tension can have both causes and repercussions that appear to be far away from your jaw. In the pages that follow, case studies will show how a wide range of conditions throughout your body can in fact be linked to TMD. This investigation will also help us to understand how the holistic practices of facial self-massage, yoga, and mindfulness can make a difference in your well-being.

⚜ 4

Dental Work and TMD

L ET'S TAKE a closer look at the repercussions—and some of the causes—
of jaw tension, beginning with your mouth. Clenching and grinding
can wear down the biting surface of your teeth over time. It can also lead
to cracked and broken teeth. Since teeth are essential to a healthy life, you
may need considerable dental work for tooth repair, including caps, crowns,
extraction, and replacement of teeth. I am reminded of a client who casually
remarked, "Teeth . . . you know, they can be replaced" when I asked whether
she was prone to clenching. I was a bit shaken by this disposable attitude
toward her body. It is true that teeth are replaceable. Dentists will never go
out of business, that is for sure. However, we might also consider that extensive dental work can be costly, painful, disruptive, and occasionally traumatic. If we want to avoid this option, we can look a little deeper and learn to
unravel the causes of jaw tension. What we discover may be surprising.

Misalignment and compression of the TMJs can permanently damage
the joints of your mouth in several ways. For starters, the disc that cushions
the movement of your jaw can get flattened out or ruptured. The ligament
that pulls this disc back while closing your mouth can lose its elasticity and
become overly stretched out. As a result, when you close your mouth, the
disc—which creates space between two pieces of bone (condyle of mandible
and saddle portion of temporal bone) cushioning the ride of your jaw—may
not be in the proper place. Eventually, the portion of your temporal bone that
forms the lovely saddle shape can flatten out from constant tension. These
changes make the act of opening and closing your mouth more difficult—

and sometimes uncomfortable, with popping, clicking, or grinding. Your jaw becomes prone to pain and even dislocation.

Root Canals and Sinusitis—Jasper's Story

While it's clear that TMD often leads to an increased need for dental work, it's worth noting that the opposite can also be true. For one client, getting his wisdom teeth removed set the stage for jaw tension and chronic sinusitis. Jasper was a big, solid guy in his mid-forties. Dressed in jeans, Doc Martens, and a punk rock T-shirt, he admitted that coming to my office was a stretch for him. However, Jasper turned out to be full of surprises. At first glance I would not have imagined him doing yoga, but he said, "My yoga teacher sent me, and I really trust her. So here I am . . . hoping you can help. Nothing else really has."

Jasper was fed up with having chronic sinus infections for most of his adult life. As I examined him, it became apparent that Jasper's upper jaw (maxillae) and cheekbones (zygomata) were jammed up, especially on the right side of his face. During one of our sessions he said, "You know, something changed after I had my wisdom teeth removed twenty years ago. That's when all this started."

While I was working to release that entrenched cheekbone, an image came into my mind of the dentist leveraging off of Jasper's face while he strained to remove those teeth. After our session, I asked Jasper about his experience with the wisdom tooth extraction. "I was out . . . but it took longer than expected, and the dentist told me it was a tough task. He said the roots went up into the sinuses and down below the jaw line." Tooth extraction can be very physical work, especially if teeth are impacted. Naturally it's impossible to know exactly what happened—but we might guess the dentist probably needed to apply significant force to remove the wisdom teeth. In his efforts to do his job, the dentist may well have leaned into Jasper's face for leverage, unknowingly compressing the facial bones. This compression could have led to Jasper's lengthy relationship with sinusitis.

The cure was to apply subtle craniosacral manipulation to decompress those bones. It was simple and effective. After a half dozen sessions, things improved dramatically: Jasper was delighted to be free of sinusitis for the first time in decades. He comes back in for a tune-up every year or so, when he notices he's been clenching and things are starting to get uncomfortable again.

Compression causes the maxillae to lose their normal cranial motion. This impediment of the inner tide means that phlegm isn't cleared from the sinuses. As you recall, the maxillae are hollow—there is a cavity, or sinus, within the bone. Small drainage holes allow phlegm to enter and exit. If your upper jawbones do not have proper cranial motion, your sinuses may not drain as they should. This can lead to sinus infections. To use an analogy from nature, what happens to a stagnant pool of water? Without movement, water is more prone to bacterial growth. This is akin to your sinuses filled with phlegm that can't drain. We can take this analogy a little further. What happens when the root of a tree finds its way into a pool of fetid water? The tree itself can become contaminated and may eventually die as a result.

Jasper's dentist noted that the roots of his wisdom teeth had entered his sinuses. This is actually pretty common. If you are prone to chronic sinus infections and the root of a tooth finds its way into the sinus cavity, this can lead to the root becoming infected. A root canal may be needed to clean it up. If the infection spreads to the tooth itself, it could require extraction.

Going Beyond Your Mouth: Shoulders and Jaws— Moshe's Story

Sometimes dental work creates a chain reaction resulting in jaw tension and discomfort elsewhere in the body. I began working with Moshe when he was six years old. When he turned nine, he got braces—and developed a nervous tic that caused his left shoulder to jump up and down erratically. The first time I saw it happen I was rather alarmed. Moshe was a good-natured, affable kid; when I asked whether the tic bothered him, he simply said, "No, not really," and rolled his eyes as his shoulder did jumping jacks. Moshe was inherently restless, so he wanted me to tell him stories nonstop while he lay on my table. It's not always easy for my storytelling brain to work alongside my client-treatment mind. So to buy time, I asked him lots of questions, with good long pauses for his answers. And then periodically we would take wiggle breaks for him to squirm around a bit, have a sip of tea, and do some stretches with me. Moshe would always settle down quite a lot over the course of the session, occasionally falling asleep. His mother was fascinated to see this. Evidently he's not a napper and tends more to be highly wired than chilled out.

Working with Moshe's body, I found that tension was building up in his jaw and being transferred to his neck. Since I had worked with him from a young age, and in particular before he had braces and an expander, it was clear the tension increase was related to the dental work. We knew enough about his life to rule out other possibilities. The effort to move teeth and reorganize Moshe's mouth was activating his trapezius, especially on the left side. After a few weeks of craniosacral the tic was greatly reduced, happening only when Moshe was under stress.

Moving teeth and reorganizing the mouth with braces and other dental interventions involves applying significant force over time. The body's reaction to these forces can be held in the tissues of the body, causing chronic muscle tension that can last for decades. While Moshe's body showed cause and effect very quickly, many times we don't see the repercussions of dental interventions for many years. I've seen the results of dental interventions on a wide range of children and adults. There's no doubt your mouth is connected to the rest of your body, and the tissues remember everything that happens to them. In the words of renowned trauma researcher Bessel van der Kolk, *the body keeps the score.*[1]

I have also seen this in my own body. I wore braces from eleven until thirteen. In my early twenties I had a considerable amount of neck tension. This was eventually resolved through yoga, craniosacral, and other modalities. Since there is no other immediate explanation, I have often wondered if the tension resulted from those two years of extensive dental work.

Guzay's Theorem—Your Jaw and Your Neck Are Closer Than You Think

So how can we understand the migration of tension in Moshe's body (and my own) from mouth to neck to shoulders? In 1976 the engineer Casey Guzay published a series of papers titled "Quadrant Theorem" in the journal *Basal Facts*.[2] Guzay was working with the Denture Research Group of Chicago to help refine and effectively illustrate the functional motion of the human jaw in keeping with the laws of physics. His work, popularly called Guzay's theorem, demonstrated that the fulcrum for your jaw's movement lies behind the TMJ. Since the temporomandibular joint is not a simple hinge joint but rather a more sophisticated structure that also enables gliding, the true axis for the jaw is between the top two vertebrae of your neck.[3] While your lower jaw may seem far away from your neck, these two parts of your body are continually influencing one another. *If there is jaw tension, there is neck tension, and vice versa.*

To get a sense of this in your own body, gently place your index and middle fingers on the back of your upper neck, just below your head. Open and close your mouth several times. Can you feel movement under your fingers? The movement is small. If you press too heavily you may not perceive it. You can also try doing this on a friend as it may be easier to perceive on someone else. The connection between the TMJs, lower jaw, and neck is important to remember, as it has far-reaching implications. Every time the mouth opens and closes, it affects the upper neck. Your neck and jaw are inextricably intertwined. *This fact plays an important role in our yoga program.*

The top vertebra of your spine, called *atlas*, lets you nod your head up and down. Atlas is named for the Greek god who bears the world on his shoulders. Indeed, sometimes your head can feel a tremendous weight when the brain within begins generating a steady stream of miserable thoughts about the burden of our worldly lives. Just below atlas lies the second vertebra, appropriately called *axis*: it allows you to turn your head right and left. Atlas

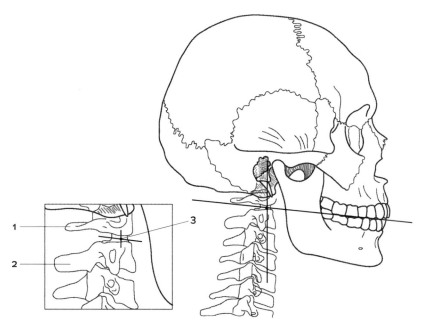

Figure 4.1: Fulcrum of mandibular motion. Guzay's quadrant theorem demonstrates the impact of biting falls behind the TMJs, between the dens of c2 and c3.

1. atlas   **2.** axis   **3.** dens

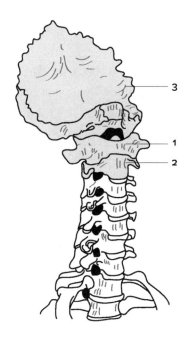

Figure 4.2: Occipital triad.

1. atlas (c1) **2.** axis (c2) **3.** occiput form a triad of interaction

and axis have complementary shapes and are quite literally intertwined. Atlas is slightly broader, while axis is slightly narrower, with a pivot post extending upward to guide the movement of atlas. Together these two vertebrae facilitate the tremendous range of motion available to your head.

Atlas and axis are very close to the base of your skull. Structurally and energetically, it is difficult to separate these parts of your body. The combined forces of aging, gravity, and muscular tension contracting your upper neck and head only make this more so. Throw in a car accident or two and it's hard to know where your head ends and your neck begins. In contrast, have you ever noticed how a young child's head seems to rest lightly atop their body, almost as if floating there? Looking back at the bones of the cranial base, we can see some interesting dynamics. First, we can see how jaw tension will impact the entire lower portion of your head—mandible, maxillae, temporals, occiput, and upper neck. It's no wonder headaches, sore necks, and back pain are often associated with TMD. We can also notice how the temporal bones may be getting pressure from both the front and back of the head. A tight and imbalanced jaw creates a tight and imbalanced neck.

Returning to Moshe's story, it's clear how changes to his mouth from orthodontia would have an impact on his neck. Since we already know that no one has a perfectly balanced body, it makes sense that one side would be affected more than the other. Returning to the important muscles we learned about, we can appreciate how jaw tension led to neck tension led to a tight trapezius on one side. Here are a few other ways that Guzay's theorem helps us to comprehend the migration of symptoms from TMD to elsewhere in your body. On a simple daily level, if you clench your teeth during the night, you are likely to wake up with a tight or stiff neck. Or if you are in a car accident and sustain whiplash, your upper neck will tighten up. If this tension is not released, in time it can migrate from your neck to your jaw causing jaw tension and TMD.

The Value of Dental Work

Despite the fact that dental work can have repercussions elsewhere in your body, it is not bad to go to the dentist. In many cases dental work is valuable and even indispensable. There is little question it is necessary for your upper and lower teeth to line up. So the issue is not one of eliminating dental corrections but rather exploring how they can be performed in ways that result in less trauma. One possibility is for more dentists to work hand in hand with cranial practitioners. At some dentist offices, a cranial practitioner is on-site, adjusting patients before and after procedures. Others provide direct referrals. Another option is for dentists to acknowledge the depth of possible impact from their work, creating an environment that mitigates potential trauma and advocates for patients' holistic well-being.

Proper tooth alignment (occlusion) lays a foundation for our overall health and well-being on many levels. Chewing is the first step in healthy digestion, preparing food to be broken down by the stomach. If teeth are out of balance, biting, chewing, and swallowing will be out of balance, and there can be repercussions far beyond the mouth. Poor tooth alignment will also throw off the alignment of the upper and lower jawbones (maxillae, temporals, and mandible). This will in turn influence other bones of the face and skull and can extend into the rest of the body.

One of my cranial teachers told the story of a famous basketball player who had unexplained knee pain. Knees are extremely important when your livelihood is made by running around an indoor court while trying to jump and throw a ball accurately into an eighteen-inch ring that's ten feet up. And a lot of people become extremely interested in resolving the problem when you are getting paid millions of dollars to perform in front of a full arena and broadcast on prime-time TV. They tried everything, as the story goes. Finally someone asked, "Did you get any dental work recently?" Why yes, indeed, he had just had a crown replaced. A quick trip back to the dentist found the crown was off by microns. After it was filed down, the knee pain went away.

I actually had a similar experience after having a filling replaced. In my youth I was a competitive athlete and ran throughout the year, competing in both indoor and outdoor track. By the spring of my senior year of high school I had managed to damage my knees to the point where I was in chronic pain. My first couple of years in college I took it easy and intuitively healed my knees through the progression of swimming, biking, and focused weight-lifting. In adulthood I took up yoga and cultivated a very different relation-ship to my body, healing my knees entirely, among other things. Due to my earlier experiences, I remain very attuned to knee pain when it arises. When my right knee began aching nonstop a few days after the replacement of a loose filling, I thought perhaps I should have the dentist take another look. His response was, "Oh wow, that's a boulder I left on top of that filling! Let me file that down for you." And guess what? I'm happy to report the knee pain went away.

$\maltese$ 5

Your Ears and Your Jaw

I N MAMMALS, the ear canal and the TMJ are very close together.[1] This evolutionary trait has an unfortunate side effect: The proximity of chronically tight and misaligned TMJs can afflict your ears in many ways, including pain and tension, hypersensitivity to sound, loss of hearing, ringing in the ears (tinnitus), or dizziness (vertigo). Proper cranial movement enables the temporal bones to clear your ear canals. As we saw in chapter 3, there is a subtle, ongoing movement—the cranial wave—throughout waking and sleeping within all of the cranial bones. This cranial wave provides a form of circulation for the skull, organs (including the brain), tissues, and fluids. Ideally your ear canals gently coil and uncoil several times a minute with the oscillation of your cranial bones. Chronic tension or compression, as well as restrictions left over from birthing, can prevent this clearing from happening, resulting in increased frequency of infections.

Ear Infections—Katie's Story

Little Katie was an active toddler who kept pulling on her ears. She'd had five ear infections the winter before she turned two. Doctors were encouraging a surgical insertion of tubes to keep her ear canals open. Her mother wanted to try a different approach, so she made an appointment with me. Working on two-year-olds is always an interesting process. Toddlers are all about movement. It's unrealistic to expect them to be still, much less to lie down on a massage table in a stranger's office. Quite naturally they are curious about their environment, wanting to explore. I attempted to engage Katie's natural desire to know more about me and my space. After greeting each other in the reception area, Katie, her mom, and I wandered through the office, saying hi to everyone we met. We talked to the plants and looked out the window to see what was happening in the garden, discussing the butterflies landing on the flowers and the birds chirping. Our mini-tour gave Katie time to arrive and feel more at ease. Eventually we made our way into my personal office where I had created a welcoming environment by laying out a blanket on the floor picnic style, with a selection of toys waiting for her.

In order to establish safety and trust, we all played together for a while before I tried to work with her body. Eventually Katie settled down in her mama's lap, where they were enjoying a picture book. After a few minutes I began touching Katie's feet. Before doing this, I asked permission within my mind, "Would it be alright for me to touch you?" She seemed to receive this. When a child is not ready to be touched, they make no bones about it, by pulling their body away from your hands or simply getting up and walking away. Developmentally, it is extremely important to respect the boundaries that children impose regarding touch. While we as adults may be bigger and stronger, there is no wisdom in forcing a child's compliance. Instead, we can skillfully support a child's autonomy and empowerment regarding touch. To force ourselves on them—even with a healing intent—is to violate their trust, confuse their natural capacity for knowing what they do and don't want, and potentially cause trauma that can last a lifetime. We can avoid all of this by simply slowing down, paying attention, and asking permission.

Feet are usually a safe way to begin to touch someone. Somehow our feet are much less vulnerable than other parts of our bodies. When I touch a person's feet, I am actually engaging with their whole body. Simple foot contact can send a message of ease and relaxation to the entire nervous system. Body and mind start to soften. As we relax, we feel safer. This leads to a greater receptivity to healing.

Gently held, Katie's feet gave her an opportunity to get to know me in a nonverbal way. As our nervous systems entrained with one another through this first contact, I created the opportunity within my mind for a second contact. When I felt I got an inner "yes" from her, I placed my hand on her sacrum.

Sacral Bone:
Involuntary Movement of the Sacrum

The sacrum is a fascinating bone, conveying much information to those who take the time to listen closely to what it wishes to express. Your sacrum is composed of five fused bones, and just below it, three to five more fused bones compose the tailbone (coccyx). It takes about twenty-five years for your sacrum and tailbone to fully fuse. As a result, there is a lot of movement in a young child's sacrum. As we learn to stand and walk, this weight-bearing and movement contribute to the stabilization of the sacrum, as well as its growth and development—a prime example of Wolff's law that form follows function. As you might imagine, if there is misalignment or imbalance in a sacrum, it can interfere with these natural developmental stages.

The inner tide manifests in a number of ways at your tail. The sacrum is constantly changing size and shape. Similar to your cranium, the bones of your sacrum very subtly broaden and shorten, and then elongate and narrow, along with the rest of your body. Additionally, the base of your spine gently oscillates between your pelvic bones. Sacral movement is both lengthwise

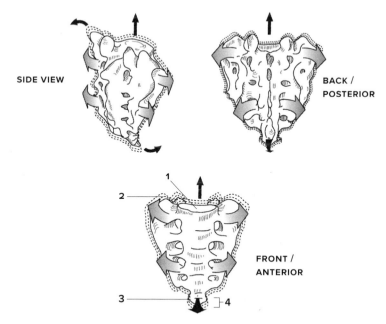

Figure 5.1: Sacrum anatomy and motion. The sacrum "breathes," subtly expanding and releasing with the inner tide. Arrows indicate the inhalation phase.

1. sacral base   **2.** lumbosacral articular surface   **3.** apex of sacrum   **4.** coccyx (tailbone)

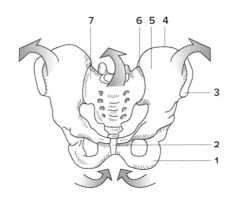

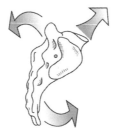

Figure 5.2: Tidal motion of sacrum in pelvis. The pelvis and sacrum have complimentary tidal motion. Restrictions in this cause pain, discomfort, and dysfunction. Arrows indicate inhalation.

1. ischial tuberosity	3. anterior superior iliac spine (ASIS)	4. iliac crest	6. sacro-iliac (si) joint
2. pubis symphysis		5. ilium (pelvic bone)	7. sacrum

and sideways, constantly balancing the many forces at play in your body and mind. This is a very strategic bone—it's all about safety and stability. Next time you are having a conversation with someone, put your awareness in your sacrum and notice how it makes continual micro-adjustments to get the best angle on the situation.

Fascial Connections

With Katie, my intention was to identify what was happening on the inside of her body, in particular with the dural tube and the reciprocal tension membrane (RTM). The dural tube is a thick membrane surrounding your spinal nerves (*dura*). It attaches at the base of your skull and ends at the second sacral segment—and it's otherwise free from any attachments within your spinal column. This pelvis-head connection is called the *core link* (figure 5.3).[2]

This head to tail connection enables us to perceive and free up the entire length of the spine by simply contacting one end. The dural tube is continuous with the reciprocal tension membrane as well as the fasciae surrounding and protecting your brain (called *meninges*, figure 5.4). The RTM holds and supports your brain like a hammock or tent, within which your brain can abide safely and comfortably.

When frequent ear infections occur, restrictions or rigidity in these membranes can be a culprit. The immobility may well be residual tension from birth. Tight membranes can limit the tidal motion that would otherwise maintain health. Katie accepted my hand on her back, and I was able to feel a tightness in the membranes associated with the movement of the temporal bones inside her head. Working with her sacrum, I invited the possibility of clearing this. Katie's sacrum responded willingly, unwinding as I simply held it with the light pressure of a cranial contact. To get a sense of this, imagine a weight of a sheet of paper resting on your body. That's about the same as the pressure of a craniosacral hold.

Eventually I placed one hand on the back of Katie's head while keeping the other on her sacrum. After a few minutes there was more fluidity in the

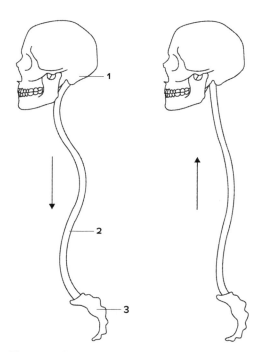

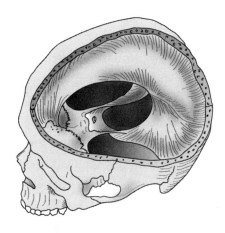

Figure 5.4: Reciprocal tension membrane (RTM) and dural twist. Membranes of the skull support the brain and are continuous with the dural tube and fascia of the body.

Figure 5.3: Core link. The dura provides a direct link (superhighway) between head and tail.

1. occiput   **2.** dural tube   **3.** sacrum spinal dura, her sacrum was moving freely, and the connection between her hips and head was more easily perceived, meaning there was less blockage within Katie's body. Noticing she was still at ease with my touch, I placed my hands softly over her ears. Sure enough, her temporal bones were blocked up. I tried to imagine how this might feel. No doubt it was uncomfortable for her. Sometimes children with blocked eustachian tubes will resist being touched on their ears for this very reason. And other times, as was the case with Katie, they actually place their hands on top of mine and press them more firmly onto their head, as if to say, "Yes, that's it, you've found the right spot! That feels good. Thank you." At the same time, Katie looked up at me, as if in surprise. We made eye contact, and I talked about what was happening. She became very quiet and still. This lasted for several minutes. And then, as if nothing had happened, she was back to being a bouncing bubbling two-year-old in constant motion. The inner tide had pushed its way through, allowing the temporal bones to regain their gentle oscillation.

Ear Canal Movement

The next step was to work inside Katie's mouth to provide a direct release to the ear canals. Ideally eustachian tubes coil and uncoil several times a minute through the tidal movement of the temporal bones. This motion supports a few different functions. The tubes equalize air pressure between the middle and outer portions of your ear while also clearing fluid and cellular debris from the middle ear. When the temporals are jammed up, the tidal motion is restricted—interfering with the clearing of the ear canals.

The eustachian tubes open directly into the far upper back of your mouth. A manual release can be provided by gently putting a gloved finger in the mouth and tapping on the tubes' openings, stimulating them to open and clear. However it's not always easy to convince a two-year-old to open their mouth and let your finger in. After demonstrating on myself and mama, we won Katie's interest and were rewarded with the chance to tap on the ear canal opening. Her ears responded well to the treatment, and it proved to be a real turning point for her health and well-being. I saw Katie regularly that winter, and she had no ear infections. Her mother was incredibly grateful to avoid the surgical implantation of tubes.

Tinnitus—Sam's story

Sam, who goes by the pronouns they/them, came to see me after a slip and fall injury that resulted in a sinus infection that knocked them flat. Dressed in overalls and a T-shirt, I might have guessed they were a construction worker. And yes, Sam did do the occasional renovation as a moonlighting gig. But in fact they loved their day job as an ASL translator. Sam had a compact, solid body with a neck like a brick. A long history of clenching and grinding most certainly contributed to that solid neck. It may have played a role in the mild, chronic tinnitus they lived with as well. A nonstop talker, Sam was full of story after story. Bright, bustling energy was their strong suit . . . Sam was a bit of a pistol. One December afternoon, Sam slipped and fell on a patch of ice, hitting the right side of their forehead on the pavement. After that came a heavy-duty sinus infection, keeping them in bed for a full month—and then the tinnitus increased dramatically. They came to see me in February.

Within a minute or two of lying down on my table, Sam's head began to call for my attention, saying, "Me first! I need your help." And so I started there. Carefully placing my hands under Sam's head, I noticed considerable tension at the back left side. Due to fluid dynamics within the head, a constriction frequently occurs opposite of where a blow happens. I sat with Sam's head resting in my palms for quite a while, allowing the fluid, membranes, brain, and skull to release. Just holding here with steady attention allowed things to start coming back into balance.

While holding Sam's head, I observed a several things. Initially Sam was a bit restless and agitated. It was hard for them to settle down. Their head didn't fully rest, as though it needed Sam to hold it up even when lying down. Inviting Sam to place their hands on their belly, below the navel, and take a few slow, deep breaths seemed to make a difference. Not long afterward, the steady stream of chatter coming from Sam stopped in mid-sentence. Then I heard a few snores. Their head turned slowly to one side. All of a sudden Sam said, "Ouch! That really hurts!" yet my hands had not moved but were simply placed under their head, which was now fully resting. At that very moment Sam had experienced a flashback of the fall. It played out through their mind and body in vivid detail. And then moments later, the tension fully released from Sam's head and neck. As trauma unravels from the nervous system and we deeply relax, it can happen that the original pain and memory of the experience return briefly as a part of the release. If we are aware and do not confuse the present with the past, this is actually a very beneficial healing process. It's like the incident is being removed from our visceral memory, the slate is wiped clean. The body can return to a state of freedom.

The blow to the head had jammed up Sam's maxillae (upper jawbones), temporal bones (ear bones), base of the skull (occiput), and upper neck— obstructing the cranial motion that clears phlegm and leading to Sam's lengthy sinus infection. This was on top of an already tight neck and jaw from years of clenching and grinding. Prior hearing loss, coupled with clenching and grinding, made Sam more vulnerable to tinnitus—which, after their experience of falling on that patch of ice, worsened to the point of being almost unbearable. Once the original head trauma was released, we began to work with the chronic tension in their neck, jaw, and shoulders. After that, there was a dramatic reduction in tinnitus, although it didn't go away entirely. I kept encouraging Sam to preserve the hearing they had left. While they told me a story about doing an intensive remodel to flip a house, I tried to plant a seed by asking, "Are you wearing ear protectors?" "Oh yeah, right . . . maybe next time."

Interestingly, as we worked together on Sam's tinnitus, they commented, "You know, when I was on vacation, the ringing completely disappeared. I was really struck by that. And it was windy on Galápagos—usually wind makes the whole thing worse. Then on the plane ride home, there it was again . . . it started right back up. What do you think of that?" Yes, indeed, what does one think of such a story?[3] This was not the first time I had heard something like this. If you think about it, it's not really all that surprising. Have you ever experienced symptoms disappearing while on vacation? The role of stress in our daily lives is an important factor in our health and well-being. When we are working and living our day-to-day life, it can be hard to maintain the same ease we might feel on vacation when we give ourselves time to relax and enjoy doing nothing.

On the energetic level, tinnitus can represent a feeling of "I don't want to hear it!" It can be helpful to investigate this question: What do you not want to hear? My client Peter was a corporate litigation lawyer. He described the time his tinnitus reached a fever pitch: "It was my last case before retirement. The case was due to go to court before a jury. The thing is, juries can be very difficult to read. I just remember how stressful it was preparing for that case . . ." You can imagine Peter's anxiety, and his mind being split between so many things. The jury, his client, the anticipated retirement . . . "How much longer do I have to carry on with this level of stress before I can *let go*?" I always wondered if he really did not want to hear one more case. Emotionally, he was "done."

Your Ears and Nervous System Regulation

The researcher Stephen Porges has noted the middle ear muscles are linked to the vagus nerve (cranial nerve X).[4] This nerve also controls the muscles of vocalization, facial expression, heart rate, and breathing. When we experience fear or anxiety, the middle ear muscles lose their tone and our capacity for hearing changes. When our primal fight-or-flight nervous system response kicks in, we become more attuned to low-frequency sounds evolutionarily associated with predators and have difficulty hearing human voices, which are of a higher frequency. Have you ever suddenly become absorbed in the hum of the refrigerator or the sound of a dog barking a mile away while not being able to hear the person sitting next to you? Our capacity for hearing plays such an important role in our survival as a species that it's hardwired into the primitive nervous system. In fact, hearing is the last sense we lose as we die. How your ears feel at any given moment can be a reflection on your experience of safety. When we feel threatened, the inner ears tend to close up, feeling tight and hard. Sometimes it's as if you have gravel in your ears. They may feel sore or as though the inner ear is jagged and uneven. They may pop or it may simply be difficult to hear. For some, this change in the ears can trigger tinnitus. At other times, when we don't feel immediately threatened, the inner ears may feel somewhat open and, if you're very sensitive, oval in shape. And when you are deeply at ease, feeling safe, your inner ears open up more fully and feel round.

Tinnitus is a tricky condition. There is no consistently successful treatment for it. In San Francisco, I receive referrals from two tinnitus clinics. Sometimes cranial work is effective, but not always. In my experience, it is rare for tinnitus to be purely physical. There are often emotional and stress-related components to the condition. Tinnitus can be dispiriting and isolating, even to the point of people becoming suicidal. In 2021 this painful reality was brought to prominence through the tragic death of the founder and CEO of the Texas Roadhouse restaurant chain, Kent Taylor. Taylor suffered from tinnitus as a lingering postacute COVID-19 symptom; its severity drove him to commit suicide.[5] If you are suffering from tinnitus, please know there are resources available for you. A psychologist I know developed a specialty of working with tinnitus through mindfulness practice, helping people to shift their relationship to their experience. In fact, if you saw the Oscar-winning film *The Sound of Metal*,[6] you may have noticed the application of awareness techniques in helping the star of the film, fictitious drummer Ruben Stone (played by Riz Ahmed) cope with his tinnitus.

Vertigo—Mary's Story

Mary's husband drove her to her first appointment. She had been in bed for the better part of two weeks, unable to work, drive, or leave her house on her own because the world began to spin whenever she sat up. MRI, CT scan, x-rays, and traditional medical exams revealed nothing. When Mary and I talked about her condition, I grew curious as to whether she had recently experienced a blow to her head or been in an accident. Indeed, about a month before the vertigo started she had been out bicycling with her family. They turned a sharp corner and she ran into a fence. While her head did not hit anything, her body lurched over the handlebars, with her head first following and then leading, as her bike came to an abrupt stop. That was enough to cause whiplash.

Whiplash

Classically understood to be a strong forward and backward movement of your head—like that of cracking a whip—whiplash can occur from just a single extreme movement. A key factor is the rapid change of direction of your body. Another important piece is the surprise factor. Mary had been pedaling along, and then her momentum was halted by the fence she didn't see and definitely hadn't anticipated. It was a big surprise. Such a sudden stop doesn't give your nervous system time to adjust, leading to a trauma response like the freezing of your body's tissues. Usually there is some level of shock that results, which can make it difficult to fully care for ourselves. These forces can quickly become compressed into our being, with compensations developing rapidly from your mind's need to cope with the situation and carry on.

Mary had a twenty-year habit of clenching, which laid a foundation for chronic muscle tension. Add to this that she had been under significant work stress for many months, and the deck was stacked. Then, right after the bike accident, Mary got poison oak that quickly spread over her entire body. Since she had a history of sensitivity to the plant, she requested steroids to treat it. Her doctor happened to be out of town, and the covering physician gave her a much higher dose than she normally took. I began to wonder whether the steroids put Mary's nervous system into a fight-or-flight, high-alert cascade. That could have been the factor that pushed things over the top, knocking her already tense structure just that micron more out of alignment enough to cause the vertigo. Her head was already in a precarious position from built-up tension over many years. Remember Guzay's theorem from chapter 4? That would be at play here: neck and jaw both tightly wound, resulting in the loss of the inner tide.

As I worked with Mary's head, I found that her upper neck was very tight and her ear bones (temporals) were stuck. Our sense of balance comes from our inner ears and upper neck. If one or both temporal bones become jammed against the other bones and lose their cranial motion, this can bring on vertigo. Inviting the cranial wave back into these areas gave Mary immediate relief. While her dizziness wasn't yet fully resolved, she could stand and walk on her own for the first time in weeks. After just a few more sessions Mary was able to go back to work, although bouts of vertigo still occurred. The bones making up the base of her head—including the skull base (occiput), ear bones (temporals), sphenoid bone (behind the eyes), and top two vertebrae of her neck—all remained under stress, with greater tension on the right side. We continued working together regularly, and during treatment we would talk about the stressors in her life. Mary revealed that, while she loved parts of her job, workplace dynamics were activating traumatic memories from a time of instability in her early childhood, caused by her alcoholic father. She had the courage and wisdom to accept the emergence of these memories as a growth point rather than a detriment. She understood that her office situation was simply playing out a dynamic that had had an impact on her, but it was not the true cause of how she felt. She kept working on her emotional and psychological well-being, as well as coming to see me once or twice a month.

A year later Mary was fully recovered. Our work together relieved the tension on her TMJs, neck, and sphenoid bone, balancing her craniosacral system throughout her body. During the course of her vertigo, Mary took a step back and considered how she could create more balance in her life. Yoga and meditation practices provided tools for stress reduction and self-reflection, allowing her childhood wounds to heal. Through mindful self-reflection Mary was able to change her relationship to some of the demands of her job so they caused her less stress. Through creative thinking and teamwork she changed other aspects of her job so they better suited her personality. She grew more fully into herself during this time. I was impressed by Mary's willingness to listen to her own being and make positive change. At times physical symptoms or illness are an expression of overwhelm and exhaustion. If we are willing to receive the message, it can also be a healing journey.

6

Headaches, Stress, Trauma, and TMD

MANY TMD SUFFERERS share a common complaint: headaches—albeit with a surprising range of symptoms and locations. Whether it's burning at the top of your head, pressure on the sides, tingling in your face, or a painful neck and jaw, it's all some form of ache in the head. Not everyone who clenches gets head pain, but many do. As you might imagine, this diversity of expression makes headaches difficult to define and fully understand. This is not a simple subject. And yet we can explore some of the ways that TMD and headaches overlap. Headaches have many causes, including tight muscles, body posture, injury, structural misalignment, biochemistry, stress, trauma, and difficult emotions. The energetics of headaches include a feeling of being under pressure. As one client said, "I just always feel as though my head is in a vise." Being "all in one's head" also applies. When we feel overwhelmed, becoming "paralyzed" and withdrawing to a safe place inside our head can happen faster than we realize. *Paralyzed* does not always mean we are incapable of action. But we may no longer be feeling ourselves. I am reminded of a client named Rossana. At some point in our work together it became apparent that the ache she felt at the back of her head was her "escape hatch." When things got overwhelming, her vulnerable inner child would be screaming, "Get me out of here!" That's when the throbbing would start. At that point, her threshold for distress had been reached. She could no longer feel the rest of her body. The torment of her head was all she knew.

One of most common types of headache associated with jaw tension is the tension headache, which begins with tight muscles. The four primary muscles of mastication (lateral and medial pterygoids, masseter, and temporalis, figures 2.8a, 2.8b), as well as sternocleidomastoid and trapezius (figures 2.9a, 2.9b), are big players here. All of these were discussed in chapter 2. Let's take a closer look at the involvement of these fellows in head pain.

Tension Headache—Penny's Story

When Penny came to see me, she had been in a lot of pain in a lot of ways for a long time. She began having terrible headaches early in the year. Then a much needed hip replacement in the spring kept her away from the physical activity she loved, particularly cycling, running, and yoga. As a result of the chronic pain, she was on disability leave from her job as a librarian and feeling a bit isolated. Additionally she was grieving the loss of her father, who had passed away the previous year. Her mother had died when Penny was in her twenties. Now in her later fifties, Penny felt acutely aware of being an orphan of sorts, with both parents gone. She was struggling with the loss of family that many of us experience at some point in our lives. Consumed by physical and emotional challenges, she was battling depression.

Besides tension headaches, Penny suffered from osteoarthritis in her neck. At times she could barely turn her head. Years of clenching likely contributed to her condition. Masseter, temporalis, and trapezius were team members in her agony. And Penny's sternocleidomastoid muscles (SCMs) in particular were very tight. When the SCMs are unyielding, over time they can actually change the shape of the upper neck, forcing it to lose its curve. A flattened cervical spine is chronically compressed and much less resilient. Her headaches radiated up over the top of her head, which spoke to the lesser and greater occipital nerves getting pinched at the base of her skull.

We could decrease Penny's suffering during sessions in my office, but between visits something would often cause her neck to seize up again. The distress would be unremitting until she came back to see me. During a chat about self-care, Penny remarked that she really loved Savasana (figure 11.24), the resting pose that comes at the end of most yoga classes. I encouraged her to try adding a body scan meditation to her Savasana—and to do it frequently, even several times a day. Why not take this time on disability as a chance to do more focused healing? Mindfulness of the body is one of the best ways to support overall relaxation. I also advised taking short mindful breaks throughout the day to simply breathe and notice how she was feeling for a few minutes at a time. I was hopeful that increasing awareness of her body and mind in daily activities would help Penny to stay closer to her emotional experience as it ebbed and flowed from dawn until dusk.

One day Penny said, "I wanted to watch the basketball game on TV. It sounds like such a simple thing, but you know, it's amazingly complicated. You have to find the right remote, switch from the TV to an app, scroll through all the options, find the event you're looking for. . . . I felt myself getting really frustrated. I am pleased to say I didn't fly off in a rage like I might have in the past, which is a good thing. And I kept talking to my wife throughout, trying to stay upbeat . . . but I felt my neck stiffening up anyway. It's been tight ever since."

Penny's body-mind awareness was awesome! I was impressed to hear how well she was tracking her emotions and body experience. How could she go that next step and prevent building up tension in her body by actually releasing the stress as it arose? We brainstormed about ways she might switch up her relationship to her experience. "What if you play with it all?" I suggested. "Try growling and grumbling and moving your body around so that you stay connected to the anger without letting it build up. Maybe you can let it out viscerally while using humor to acknowledge how you are feeling. *Acting it out* is more fun than 'acting out' with anger. You're less likely to unintentionally hurt your partner—or yourself—if you are moving your body instead of allowing tension to build up from suppressing your emotions." A slow smile spread across Penny's face. She seemed to like the idea of growling her way through her frustration.

The Role of Stress

Stress and headaches are intimate partners. The same is true with stress and jaw tension. One might even say these factors form an unholy trinity of sorts. If we remove stress, the symptoms of headaches and jaw tension go way down. And yet not everyone who gets stressed will clench or have headaches. That is why it's helpful to look at the underlying factors that can contribute to jaw tension. As Kelly McGonigal, author of *The Upside of Stress*,[1] astutely recognizes, "A meaningful life is a stressful life." Stress arises when we care about something. Our caring is an expression of our humanity. It may be helpful to investigate the role stress plays in jaw tension and headaches—and in our lives.

Why Do We Clench under Stress?

The trigeminal nerve (cranial nerve V) is responsible for sensation and motor function in your face. It is the most complex cranial nerve with numerous branches. The mandibular division controls biting and chewing and is the largest branch of this essential nerve. Cranial nerve V is hardwired into your brain stem in the lower back area of your head near the skull base. Sometimes called the reptilian or old brain, the brain stem is responsible for fundamental bodily functions like breathing, heart rate, body temperature, digestion, and sleeping/waking cycles. This part of your brain sends signals to the rest of your body to activate the fight-or-flight stress response. When you are under stress, it's easy to become dysregulated. Your nervous system goes into overdrive, activating the sympathetic response to fight back or run away, even if there's nowhere to go and no one to fight. This activation can spill over into the trigeminal nerve, with your jaw being top on the list of activation due to the sheer size of the mandibular branch. From an evolutionary view, it's natural that your teeth would start gnashing in preparation to show your intimidating pearly whites in order to scare off or bite a potential predator as needed. This is an important line of defense. But for some, once the jaw starts clenching, it can be hard to stop. It can become a self-perpetuating cycle of misery. The pain from the nonstop clenching feeds back into brain stem activation that perpetuates the chomping.

The Role of Trauma

What makes something traumatic? Simply stated, trauma occurs when experience happens faster than we can integrate. Our nervous system becomes overwhelmed and specific biochemical cascades take place to facilitate our survival. But what does it feel like in your body and mind when trauma is occurring? And how can we recover from it? It can help to look at how animals respond when hunting and being hunted. As humans, we *are* animals; our instincts for survival and self-protection are fundamental to our nature. When something unexpected happens, our physiology responds systematically, attempting a series of interventions. The polyvagal theory as developed by Stephen Porges helps us to understand our instinctive responses to life's challenges, including trauma.[2] Porges has identified the vagus nerve (cranial nerve X) as a significant and fascinating player in regulating our physiological capacity to change states—including during traumatic experiences. *Poly-vagal* indicates that the vagus functions in different ways. Cranial nerve X is distinct because, while it originates in the brain stem, it has the longest pathway of all the cranial nerves, much of it outside of the head. In fact, 80 percent of the vagus provides information from the internal organs to the brain. Translated from Latin, *vagus* means "wanderer" . . . this is the nerve that wanders around your body gathering information about your experience to inform your brain as to how to act for your optimum survival. In particular, the vagus connects the internal organs, brain, and heart.

Social Engagement System

All of us have a fundamental need for safety. As a result, we are constantly checking our environment for any possible threat. For most of us, this occurs below the threshold of awareness. When a potential danger is perceived, our first line of defense is connection—Porges calls this the *social engagement system*[3] (see figure 2.7). We might view this as our face-heart connection: communicating our heart's need for love and safety through our face. Think of it this way: if you are in trouble, another person is infinitely more creative and resourceful than any object.

At an early stage of feeling threatened, the nerves involved in social connection will light up. These nerves will activate the muscles involved in creating facial expressions (to engage others), moving your eyelids (to regulate a social gaze), your middle ears (to discern human voices), your voice (so you sound appealing to others), and your jaw (for chewing or suckling). The activation of these muscles is intended to allow you to build connection to save yourself from harm. Nerves involved in turning and tilting your head also fire up, so you can look toward others and engage them through the gestures of welcome that are common to us all. These expressions and movements are all attempts at coregulation: creating safety between your nervous system and others.

In essence, your attempts to coregulate and connect with others are a lower level of activation of your nervous system. If your friendly glances and welcoming tone of voice are met with nonresponse, stone-cold stares, or perhaps even aggression, then your nervous system will ramp up to mobilize. Porges defines stress as "when your nervous system loses the capacity to coregulate in the presence of another."[4] Your stress response includes increased heart rate, lungs expanding to increase oxygen flow, and muscles tensing to run away or fight back. This is full-on sympathetic nervous system activation.

Now imagine your efforts to get away or fight are ineffective. Your opponent is much bigger, stronger, more aggressive, and perhaps there is nowhere to run to. What happens next? If the attempts to take action are futile, the nervous system shuts down. You may go limp or even pass out. Or you may simply space out, disconnecting from your body, perhaps even witnessing what happens next from a distant place. Freezing is the oldest response, hierarchically. From an evolutionary standpoint it's been working for a long time. Think of the ancient turtles who use this strategy well or possums "playing dead." The freeze response slows your breathing and heart rate considerably, which is why some lose consciousness. This is a parasympathetic stress response. Others may have an out-of-body experience. Some feel threatened, and for others it's actually strangely pleasant. Each one of us has our unique version of these responses.

Understanding Trauma—Penny's Story Continues

Early in my work with Penny I began to intuit that childhood trauma may have played a role in her headaches and depression. Her nervous system tended to be in something like a freeze state, and her love of movement and exercise hinted at a high that helped her feel a freedom she loved but couldn't settle down from afterward. In other words, it was hard for her to self-regulate. Eventually, Penny shared her trauma story with me. When she was eleven, her family moved to a town where they didn't know anyone. There was a pack of kids in the new neighborhood that played together. One day, one of the older boys from a house on the next block snuck up on her in the laundry area of someone's garage. Coming from behind, he grabbed her and pinned her to the wall while groping her body, putting his hands between her legs and fingers inside of her. He was bigger and stronger. She wanted desperately to escape, but there was no way out. What happens in the moments when we don't like what is happening to our body? When our experience is so horrifying and uncomfortable all we want is to disappear? In particular, what happens when we can't prevent someone from touching us in a way that we do not consent to?

Watching my neighbor's cat Felicia play with a mouse in my backyard,

I begin to understand the range of human responses better. Initially the mouse runs across the yard. Felicia pounces, catching it between her paws. After a few seconds, she removes her paws to reveal the mouse, sitting there, unharmed. But the mouse doesn't run away. When running didn't work, his nervous system defaulted to the oldest trick in the book, and now he's immobilized. In this case, it works; Felicia loses interest and wanders off. And then a few moments later, the mouse comes back to life and scampers across the yard, disappearing down a hole to the safety of home. But what was the experience of the mouse while it was beneath Felicia's paws? From the outside we might assume it was frozen in terror, in a high-alert state. However, this isn't always true. In freeze state both the sympathetic (arousal) and parasympathetic (sedation) systems can be activated, and it varies which one is "in charge."[5] While some people (or mice) experience fear, others are in a protected state, numb to what their body is experiencing. This dissociation can be appreciated as yet another proficient lifesaving strategy—but it creates a polarization between body and mind that needs to be bridged adroitly. The range of possible responses presents a unique challenge with regard to reintegration after trauma.

Going back to those moments when Penny was trapped by her abusive neighbor: What was going on in her body and mind? She wanted to run and couldn't. She was bullied into compliance, unable to prevent a violation. Her sympathetic nervous system's initial response was "Get away!" Adrenaline flowed, increasing her heart rate and contracting her muscles in preparation for fighting and fleeing. When it became obvious that escape was impossible, the dorsal vagal freeze response kicked in, slowing her heart rate, relaxing her muscles, and disconnecting her mind from her physical body's experience. To be very clear, this was a biological survival response. This was not a personal choice.

Later on, after Penny went home, she tried to talk about what happened—a natural and positive instinct for integrating her experience, coming out of dorsal vagal freeze state and back into her feeling body. But the situation was too upsetting for her mother, who went into denial, unable to hear her daughter's words that day or any other day. Penny was left to cope on her own. Years later, Penny recalled that her mom and dad "were great parents overall. They were thoughtful and caring. But my mom . . . ," Penny's voice trailed off. "When she found out what happened, she just shut down. So I just had to stuff it inside and carry on." Not long after this Penny began to clench. Her body-mind's intelligent survival response was to dissociate yet again, to stop feeling her emotions. This does not mean the trauma went away. Rather, it was buried below the surface, inaccessible for a period of time. A freeze response that doesn't end can lead to depression.

When we suppress our emotions, our muscles contract. Over time this becomes chronic, limiting range of motion as some muscles become overdeveloped and others weak from underuse. We feel stiff, dull, and heavy. Eventually, internal organs become depleted from the constant cycling between activation of fight-or-flight sympathetic response and shutdown of dorsal vagal freeze. Hormonal and mood dysregulation set in. Anxiety, depression, rage, and despair become normal experiences. We forget what happiness feels like. The process of reintegrating body and mind takes time. Important ingredients in the healing process can include patience, loving-kindness, compassionate connection, conscious movement, and safe touch.

Pandemic Headache—Jasmine

Jasmine started having an intense, unremitting headache on the right side of her head at the beginning of the COVID-19 pandemic. The sensation would alternate between stabbing and burning and encompass her head, neck, shoulder, and right arm. Jasmine had been clenching since she was a teenager, and headaches occasionally accompanied her menstrual cycle (along with cramps and irritability)—but nothing like this level of pain had ever happened before. A few months earlier she'd had a minor car accident; she was rear-ended while sitting at a stoplight. She'd had no immediate symptoms, but little accidents can often have a big impact on the nervous system. Problems may show up months later. I considered it to be a piece to the puzzle of Jasmine's discomfort.

A pretty, slight young woman in her mid-twenties, Jasmine wore simple clothes in muted colors, as though she didn't want to attract attention to herself. Sitting in my office, it seemed she might just disappear, blending in with the chair, the walls, and the carpet. As she moved onto the treatment table, Jasmine carefully placed her body in the very center, lined up perfectly straight, with her hands folded across her belly. Her meticulousness implied she didn't want to take up too much space. Overall her movements projected a sense of containment.

Jasmine's anxiety went way up during the pandemic. The lack of information available to everyone initially created a murky, fear-inducing situation. Jasmine—along with so many of us—was suddenly faced with the uncertainty of life. Government restrictions meant limited freedom in daily activities. Routines were upended, with habitual comforts and pleasures temporarily forbidden. Fortunately, Jasmine's job was stable and she was able to work from home most of the time, so health and income weren't much at risk. Her homelife was steady too. She lived with her boyfriend, their relationship was strong, and she felt supported by him.

Concurrent to the pandemic and head pain onset, Jasmine began having memories of physical and sexual assault from her childhood. The memories came in her dreams and centered around her father. In some way, it was difficult to discern what was real and what was imagined. She talked with her sister, who corroborated her experience of abuse from their father. She got into therapy, and her therapist referred her to me.

After a few craniosacral sessions Jasmine said, "Well, I don't hate my life anymore." My heart both broke and jumped to hear her say this, as there was clearly misery in the statement—but also hope. When I asked her why, the answer was, "Mostly what I experience now is just a burning sensation, which I can live with. It's when it gets to be the stabbing pain in my head that I want to kill myself." While touching Jasmine's body, I frequently received images of trauma. To build safety and trust I told her what I was noticing and asked about her experience. Talking mindfully about trauma can normalize it in a supportive way, overcoming the shame and stigma. After all, we have all experienced trauma; it's part of being human. Recognizing this can eliminate our sense of isolation, of feeling different, damaged, or "less than" anyone else. Trauma can be healed through conscious, compassionate connection, which allows for nervous system regulation. Traumatic memories are inherently uncomfortable. No one wants to relive agonizing past experiences. And yet flashbacks present opportunities to ameliorate the past. Trauma shows itself when we are ready to reconcile our experience, reconnect with ourselves, forgive others, and become more whole. While trauma patterns may never fully disappear, they can be integrated and understood. Held in the light of mindful awareness and loving-kindness, we can relate wisely to the painful experiences of our lives, growing and healing into a more easeful relationship with our past.

During one session I touched Jasmine's feet and an image of her desperately trying to flee from someone or something filled my senses. I described this to her, and she said, "That was definitely well within my childhood experience." Another time, as I sat with my hands under her shoulders the words, "Help me! I'm trapped!" came into my mind. What exactly did this refer to? I couldn't know for sure, but as I continued working with Jasmine, I began to wonder if the unique conditions of the pandemic were activating old trauma. Was the nebulous virus replaying the role of her father, always lurking in her life, creating a familiar feeling of instability mixed with fear of reprisal for unknown actions? If you "try on" Jasmine's experience for a few minutes, you might feel within your body the tremendous anxiety and insecurity of a child who never quite knew when her father—whom she shared a home and was dependent upon—might become her attacker and abuser. Did the restrictions imposed due to the public health crisis somehow recreate for her nervous system the childhood sense of being trapped and unable to get away from her father's grasp? And was this why a nerve became entrapped, creating a neuralgia pattern? Bodies tell stories in amazing ways. If we can turn toward our pain with receptivity and curiosity, it may be sharing something very important.

Jasmine's condition improved with each session. She was tremendously motivated to heal. In addition to practicing a body scan meditation, she enrolled in the Mindfulness-Based Stress Reduction Program at her local hospital. She began experimenting with online yoga classes as well. The benefits were undeniably apparent. Her life was less debilitated by physical and emotional distress. Gradually she grew more comfortable talking about past trauma. She started to feel more at ease with herself. Often at the end of sessions she was radiant, smiling and joking with me. However, I was most struck by the day that she walked in for her appointment and said at the beginning of the session, "I'm less consumed by the pain now. I just see it as a part of my life. I notice it, but I'm not obsessed with it anymore. Before, I would spend so much time trying to get rid of it, googling about it, trying to find cures and treatments. Now, it's just there. I can go on with my life." Her presence was lighter, she sat in a more relaxed way and seemed to take up space in the room in a way that was very pleasant. She was no longer blending with the chair, so to speak. While there is always some mystery to how, when, where, and why trauma arises, ultimately we can trust in the process that presents itself. Jasmine was wise when she sought help in coping with her memories and the agitation in body and mind she was experiencing.

Migraine and TMD

Migraine and TMD have a complex relationship. A migraine is not simply a headache but rather a neurological disorder with head pain—usually on either the right or left side but not the whole head—as a symptom. It's also very difficult to diagnose. The only way to be certain you are experiencing migraines is through a comprehensive neurological evaluation, which may be extremely helpful if you suspect you are a migraineur. Knowing what you are working with can guide you to find appropriate remedies. Eighty-five percent of migraineurs are women, although, interestingly, in childhood more boys experience them. Ninety percent of migraineurs have a family member who also suffers, which indicates a genetic component.[6] Specific genes have been identified corresponding with migraines. The field of epigenetics teaches us genes can be turned on and off, which means having the migraine genes does not make you fated to experience migraines.

The exact cause of migraines is still not fully understood. However, we do know some of what occurs, as well as what brings relief. There's some indication that the pain experienced during a migraine is coming from the meninges (the specialized fascial membranes within your head); in particular the dura mater and the falx cerebri are highly innervated.[7] Looking through the lens of physiology and biochemistry, we learn that when the amount of blood—and thus oxygen—flowing to your brain stem is dangerously low, the trigeminal nerve releases CGRP (calcitonin gene-related peptide), a neurotransmitter that relaxes blood vessel walls causing vasodilation.[8] This decreases blood pressure, thus increasing blood flow and oxygen supply.[9] Since your brain stem is essential to regulating the functions that keep you alive, this is a lifesaving measure. It can be helpful to acknowledge that while migraines are supremely uncomfortable, what you are experiencing is your body activating an important survival mechanism.

The brain receives blood from two places: the internal carotid arteries coming up the front of your neck and the vertebral arteries at the back of your head.[10] Tight sternocleidomastoids can actually influence either of these pathways, and Guzay's theorem reminds us that clenching will tighten the upper cervicals, potentially affecting the vertebral arteries. For some, migraine can be activated positionally. I have a client who realized that her pillow was too high. It put her neck at a strong angle, causing her migraines.

Positional migraine triggers like this tend to be associated with a history of neck and jaw tension, as well as stress and trauma. Hypermobility can also play a role.

Another starting point is squeezed maxillae (your upper jawbones, figure 2.4) forced to move not only upward but also backward as you clench, compressing the pterygopalatine ganglion (sometimes called the sphenopalatine ganglion).[11] This large nerve plexus is a neighbor to the maxillary portion of the trigeminal nerve, which it also connects to, via the pterygopalatine nerves. Distressed neighbors influence one another—even if they are body parts. Compression of this ganglion can start the vasodilation cascade that precedes migraine.[12] This is why a cranial technique that decompresses the upper jawbones is often effective for relieving migraines. This technique is aptly called *Sutherland's Grip*. In fact, it can be taught to clients so they can do it on themselves. Once upon a time I came upon a housemate exiting our kitchen in moderate distress. Prone to migraines, she had skipped lunch (after staying up too late the night before and drinking coffee in the morning) and felt a migraine coming on. Standing there in the kitchen entryway, we had a simultaneous maxillary bone release session as I guided her through the process. Her face brightened after a few minutes. "I think it's working," she said. "I'm getting hungry." And she returned to the kitchen to make herself lunch.

Even without knowing the biochemistry—which had not yet been discovered—Dr. Sutherland noted that early childhood head trauma could cause an imbalance in the sphenobasilar joint that would result in migraines years later.[13] Something as simple as falling head over heels down the stairs or tumbling off a bicycle could produce this, though it might not be immediately apparent upon conventional medical examination. An off-balance sphenoid bone can contribute to a variety of conditions, including scoliosis and dyslexia, and may result in neck and jaw tension over time. (Remember, the lateral and medial pterygoid muscles, figure 2.8b, attach the lower portion of your sphenoid to your jaw.)

Hormones are another factor in migraines. Your jaw is linked to your hormonal cycle through estrogen receptors in the mandible.[14] While the relationship between estrogen and migraines is experienced by many women, it isn't without ambiguity. It is possible to have normal estrogen levels but still experience cyclic headaches. Thus it seems the trigger is the *fluctuation* of hormones rather than an imbalance. Additionally, most women find that their headache patterns change for better or for worse as they enter new stages of life. Menarche, fertility, perimenopause, and full menopause can bring either an increase or decrease of migraines. There are as many types of migraine as there are migraineurs.

Setting biochemistry aside, we might look more closely at the ways in which a migraine is asking us to take care. Migraines insist that you go to bed, lie down in a dark, quiet room, and try to sleep until they pass. Your physiology has taken over and demanded the rest it needs. For some migraineurs, relaxing is really difficult. Their body may well need to hijack their mind's ambitions and create the opportunity for some downtime. For an overwrought nervous system, taking time for repose is quite possibly the best thing you could do.

In working with all manner of headaches, as well as stress, it's important to ask, *Is my life in balance?* Do you feel you have the time and space to cultivate inner well-being, share meaningful connection with others, express yourself openly, and move your body joyfully? Does your day allow for both quietude and engagement with others? Can you live contentedly, without a constant fear of insufficiency? While balance can be hard to achieve in a capitalist society, it is still worth striving for. Watch out for the ever-moving carrot of success dangling in the distance. The expectations put on us to show up, perform, achieve, and produce can become a tremendous burden. When employers expect sixty hours or more of labor each week, or when skyrocketing housing and food costs are forcing you to work more than is sustainable, it's easy to feel as though you are on a hamster wheel, relentlessly running in unsatisfying circles. Stress is the result.

Migraine and Unresolved Birth Trauma— Stephanie's Story

Stephanie came to see me when she was twenty-eight years old. Bright and vivacious, she was an aspiring filmmaker and loved her work for a nonprofit film production company. She saw the potential to change the world in good ways through film, and this social activism brought purpose and drive to her life. She often worked twelve-hour days, skipped lunch, and drank plenty of coffee. Her hard work was paying off: she had just been awarded full scholarship to a PhD film program in Texas. We began to work together frequently to try and get her ready for this transition.

Stephanie had attended a workshop with me and then came to see me seeking relief from migraines. She'd endured them daily since adolescence and was on prescription medication to help with the pain. She also had chronic jaw and neck tension and a habit of clenching. I noticed she was an avid gum chewer, a common habit for people with TMD, which unfortunately only makes your jaw tighter. After a month of weekly appointments, the jaw tension improved and her migraines were less frequent—although they were still far from gone. As we continued working and her muscles relaxed, I noticed something that was previously hidden. At the base of her skull, the occipital bone (figure 2.2b) felt rotated, and there seemed to be chronic tension inside the bone itself. It was like a spiraling tug-of-war happening within one bone.

"What do you know about your birth?" I asked. "Was there any difficulty?"

"Yes, actually," Stephanie replied. "There were challenges. I don't know the details, but there were complications and it took a very long time. I was caught in the birth canal for an extended period. My mom said it was really difficult. Eventually they used forceps to pull me out."

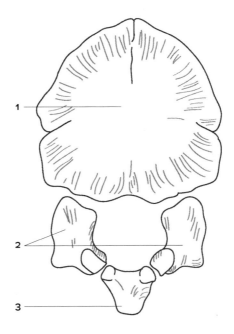

Figure 6.1: The occiput at birth. The occipital bone is in four pieces at birth:

1. squama   **2.** condyle(s)   **3.** basilar portion

Even the smoothest of births involve intense compression and rotation from the combination of contractions and the process of exiting the womb. An infant's head has to become exactly the size of the mother's pelvis to be born. To do this, skull bones will overlap. If you have ever seen a newborn's head, you may have remarked on its slightly conical shape. This usually resets itself within about three days. The compression experienced during birthing is a part of the proper unfolding, or blooming and flowering, of the skull and of the baby herself. This is part of nature's miraculous design. However, unresolved tensions can linger in the head and body of an infant—particularly if the birth was prolonged or there were complications.

The skull base (occipital bone) is in four pieces in a newborn. These pieces fuse up over a child's first five years to form the singular occiput. Even a slight misalignment between these four bones results in something called *intraosseous tension* within the cells of the mature occipital bone.[15] This is what I was sensing in the back of Stephanie's head. Imagine pieces of a puzzle that fit tightly in one area but loosely in another. The pieces that fit tightly are visibly compressed. Those that fit loosely show tiny

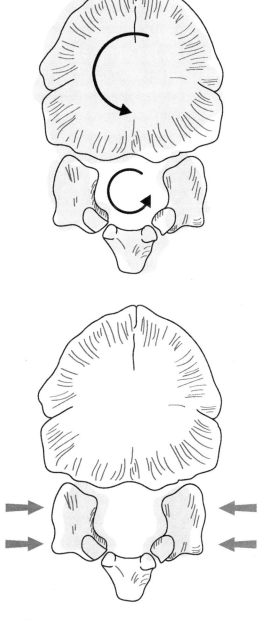

Figure 6.2: Occipital distortions. Birthing dynamics can cause tension patterns between portions of the occiput. Arrows indicate the direction of birthing forces.

gaps between them. When the pieces of the infant's skull that will form the occipital bone are misaligned, this is how they rest against one another.

A spiraling motion left over from Stephanie's birth was still held within the cells of her occipital bone. Unresolved tension of this sort is transmitted within the head and throughout the body via the reciprocal tension membrane that attaches to the occipital bone. In Stephanie's case, the result was migraines. Careful work, over time, allows tension to release from the cells. As the internal sense of tug-of-war dissipates, the cells begin to work together more harmoniously.

It's hard to know what the original cause of Stephanie's jaw tension was. And which came first, TMD or headaches? My suspicion is her difficult birth laid a foundation for the TMD that showed up later in life, like her migraines. Of course, stress and habits are always important factors too. Part of our work together was to identify any triggers to her migraines, so Stephanie began paying attention to her lifestyle choices. She cut out caffeine and started avoiding all-nighters, focusing instead on getting enough sleep, eating well, and correcting her body posture—particularly when on the computer. These changes helped Stephanie create a stabler and more sustainable way of living—a tactic that often has benefits for migraineurs. While it can be hard for any of us to accept limitations, especially when we are young, there is wisdom in learning to mindfully track ourselves throughout the day. Stop, breathe, and ask yourself, *How am I feeling now?* Then wait and listen for the answer that comes from within.

Migraines can have a very broad range of triggers, so it's extremely beneficial to take some time to learn what sets you off. All migraineurs, regardless of gender, can benefit from keeping a moon journal (page 241). Awareness of the moon's cycle reminds us to notice our own ebbs and flows. Take note of whether you've had a headache, what you've eaten, your times of sleeping and waking, and what may have happened on any given day. For women, tracking your hormonal cycle is important, including menstruation and ovulation. Frequently we can notice three triggers coming together to cause a migraine. For example, staying up late, skipping breakfast (or any meal), and being premenstrual. Or another might be being under stress at work, sitting next to someone wearing perfume, and eating something unusual. You get the idea. In general, migraines can be activated by changes in your environment (a barometric pressure drop or temperature/season change), diet (missed meals, food additives, unusual foods, caffeine, and alcohol), and lifestyle (overworking, losing sleep, inconsistent schedule). With careful observation you will learn your own unique patterns. Through knowing these, you can make wise choices.

If you are prone to any form of headache, it can be helpful to remember you have the power to decrease your discomfort and *change your relation-ship with your pain.* This will be explored more fully in parts two and three of this book. TMD and headaches are so intimate, we can't always know which is *cause* and which is *effect*. Even so, simple changes in your daily activities and working with your mind can help you heal.

⚜ 7

Hips, Feet, Hypermobility, and Your Jaw

IT CAN BE hard to believe that conditions such as sciatica, scoliosis, sacroiliac pain, fertility issues, hormonal imbalance, and digestive disorders may be linked to jaw tension. In this chapter we'll take a look at how this might happen. We'll even go all the way down to your feet. But first, here's a simple exercise to begin exploring these connections. Close your mouth and purposefully clench your teeth—make sure your upper and lower teeth are firmly touching (normally your upper and lower teeth should not touch unless you are actively chewing food. However, for the sake of this exercise, let's give it a try). Now, try to breathe into your belly. What do you experience?

TMD interferes with breathing. When you do not breathe freely, there are significant repercussions. Your breath is your simplest and most immediate nexus of health and well-being. Breathing freely equates to health. Restricted breathing is associated, over time, with ill health.[1] Muscular tension, decreased flexibility, and increased rigidity in your body are commonly associated with poor breathing. So are depression and anxiety. Less oxygen means internal organs begin to suffer, which can disturb bodily processes such as digestion and hormonal regulation. Let's take a closer look at some of the relationships between your jaw and your lower body.

Sciatica—Jane's Story

Jane contacted me just after returning from a transformational trip to Africa. She'd been on a much needed sabbatical from her beloved but stressful job running a nonprofit. The African journey was a once-in-a-lifetime, long-dreamed-of event that proved deeply heart-opening and transformational on a spiritual level. Upon her return, however, while she was walking down the jet bridge into the San Francisco airport, sciatica struck. The nerve pain running down the length of her legs was so severe that she was unable to stand, sit, or walk without support. By the time she reached out to me, Jane was on disability and unable to drive. I went to her home twice a week to try and reverse her condition quickly enough to avoid nerve degeneration. During our time together I learned she had experienced considerable childhood trauma, primarily because of her alcoholic father. The abuse included incest. She had a long history of clenching and pain in her TMJs.

As I touched Jane's body, I found that her sacrum was stuck. I sensed Jane feeling paralyzed by fear, as though she were standing on a precipice and one false move could send her over the edge. There was a disconnect between my internal experience of Jane and how she presented. Her manner was animated and engaged, so she didn't *look* fearful. I wondered if a very old trauma had been reactivated for her. I began working with her feet and hips, with the intention of supporting energy to move down and out, grounding Jane and inviting her to feel safety and connection with Mother Earth.

The sacral bone is fundamental to our capacity to stand, walk, and move on our own. It is also home to *muladhara* and *svadhisthana*, the first and second chakras. (See figure 3.2.) Muladhara represents root energy—your personal determination to survive—as well as tethering to Gaia. The second chakra, svadhisthana, is relational—including how we feel about ourselves in relationship to others and our sexual energy. Positionally, the sacrum is vulnerable to a complexity of dynamics (review figure 5.2 for the anatomy of this), from the visceral reactions of anger, fear, and vulnerability to the undulation of your pelvis as you walk, dance, play, or make love. Surrounded as it is by several big bones—including the rest of your spine, your pelvic bones, the pubic symphysis, and let's not forget the neighboring thighbones, which are the biggest, strongest bones of your body—your sacrum needs to *move*, not only as your body moves through space but also internally through the inner tide. When we do not allow our hips and sacrum to move, there are repercussions. Backache, headache, neck pain, and instability in the legs and pelvis are all well within the range of possible reactions to a stiff sacrum. And, of course, there is sciatica.

Jane's sacrum responded fairly well to craniosacral treatment; she was able to stand and walk short distances after just a couple of sessions. But she still felt uncomfortable driving and lacked the stamina to resume work. Likewise her sacrum wasn't quite willing to fully let go yet. After only two weeks—which some might consider a bit impatient—Jane said, "I've plateaued. I don't seem to be getting any better. Is there anything else we can do?" Actually, there *was* another approach I had considered . . . but I had hesitated due to Jane's history of oral trauma. It involved accessing the pelvis-head connection—the core link—through her mouth.

Up to that point, we'd worked directly with Jane's pelvic floor. An imbalanced pelvic floor, with either tight or overstretched and unstable muscles, can cause sciatica pain by either trapping (in the case of tightness) or aggravating (in the case of overstretching) the nerve. This is because the sciatic nerve passes between the piriformis and coccygeus muscles of your pelvic floor (at least in most people; about 15 percent of the time it bifurcates, or goes right through, the piriformis muscle).[2]

But there are other ways to access the pelvic floor. Techniques inside of the mouth to release the lateral pterygoid muscle (figure 2.8b) can effectively release the pelvic floor—when you have formed the trust and safety necessary to perform this work. I was hopeful this might do the trick, but with Jane's past oral trauma, it was important to proceed with caution. We talked about how she might feel about this approach and how to help her feel secure. Through careful communication between us, with space for expressions of tears, anger, rage, and grief, Jane was able to receive this modality and experienced immediate relief. Soon after, she was able to pick up the threads of her life with renewed energy, no longer in constant pain.

Sometimes transformation needs help moving all the way through the physiology. We may see where we need to go next but not be quite ready to fully embody our new reality. The body may require support, catching up to the mind's idea. And perhaps there are strong emotions seeking release on your journey from vision to actualization.

Head to Tail Connection: Core Link

As we noted in chapter 5, your head and your tail (sacrum) are coupled by the dural tube, a thick, fibrous membrane surrounding your spinal nerves and brain (figure 5.3). When a nerve leaves the spinal column, it is wrapped in dura for protection. Once out of the spinal column, the dura is called *fascia* and becomes a part of the connective tissue membrane system of your

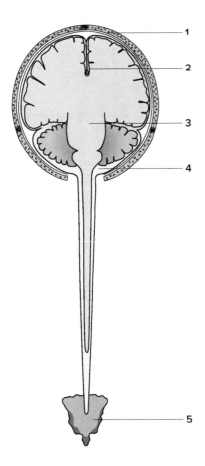

Figure 7.1: Parts of the Craniosacral System.

1. Mobility of the cranial bones
2. Reciprocal tension membrane
3. Motility of the central nervous system
4. Fluctuation of CSF
5. Involuntary motion of the sacrum between the ilia

body. The dura and fascia are continuous and composed of similar materials despite having different names and locations.[3] Within your spine, the dural tube attaches at the *foramen magnum* (opening at skull base) as it leaves your head and then flows freely until it reattaches at your sacrum.[4] The attachments at top and bottom provide a direct connection to either end of your spine. The cranial wave transmits via this tube as a rhythmic ripple. Because the dura is fairly inelastic, restricted movement patterns are broadcast from head to hips with liquid-lightning speed. Think of the dural tube as a superhighway of information, transmitting subtle movement patterns and restrictions from your head to your tail. Dr. Sutherland, in his early craniosacral research, named this inner superhighway the *core link*[5] in recognition of its importance. Just as Guzay's theorem reminds us of the jaw-neck reciprocity, the core link demonstrates the association between your neck and hips.

Imagine the spine as a delicate strand of beads. Movement or lack thereof at one end affects the other end. If the top end is restricted, then the bottom will also have limited movement. To get a sense of this, hold one end of a strand of beads between two fingers, letting the other end hang free. Gently twitch the end between your fingers. What happens to the other end?

You may notice that the loose end makes a larger movement. That is to say, it moves at a larger amplitude. This is very similar to your spine. The beads between your fingers are like the top of your spine where it meets your head. The end that hangs freely is like your sacrum. The gentle movement you created represents the inner tide. A minute adjustment to your cranial bones can have a large impact at your sacrum, because that's where the amplitude of the inner tide is the greatest and most easily perceived. Jane's story demonstrates this very well. We got some relief by working at her sacrum. We got much more relief by working at her head. At the same time it was important to address her hips first, precisely because there is more movement there. Releasing her sacrum directly helped to establish stability.

Three Mothers and Reciprocal Tension: The Dural Tube

The dural tube is composed of three layers of fascia within your head and spinal column. *Pia mater*, the delicate innermost layer, lays directly on your brain and spinal nerves, providing a fluid barrier. Translated from Latin, the name means "tender mother." The middle layer, *arachnoid mater*, named for its spiderweb-like appearance, is the most elastic. *Dura mater*, the outermost and thickest layer of membrane that protects your brain and spinal nerves, translates as "tough mother." What a lovely image this creates for our minds. Three tender, supple, and fierce mothers shielding your brain and spinal nerves, parts of your body so essential to your well-being.

Inside your head, these three layers provide a sophisticated support system for your brain to maintain homeostasis. Cerebrospinal fluid flows between pia and arachnoid mater, continually bathing, nourishing, and cleansing your brain at the perfect temperature. Dura mater separates into two layers and forms membranes, the *falx cerebri* and the *tentorium cerebelli*, which suspend your brain, making it very stable no matter how you choose to move your body on the outside. Even when you go upside down, your brain remains buoyant. The falx cerebri runs vertically from your forehead to the back of your head, separating the right and left hemispheres of your brain. It begins at your ethmoid bone (above your nose and between your eyes), runs up the center of your frontal bone and along the suture between the parietal bones at the top of your head, and ends at your occipital bone. The tentorium cerebelli runs horizontally, separating upper and lower portions of your brain (cerebrum and cerebellum). Beginning at the clinoid process of your sphenoid bone, it attaches to the temporal bones at the sides of your head—and a little on the parietal bones as well—and ends at the occipital bone at the back of your head.

The attachment sites are important: this is where the pulling of imbalanced membranes is felt most strongly. The tension from this pulling can have widespread impact. Within the head it can force cranial bones to lose their rhythmic oscillation, causing headaches, disrupted brain function, and other phenomena. The falx and the tentorium interface most directly at the back of your head, forming a tent of sorts where they both attach at your occipital bone. Together, they create the *reciprocal tension membrane* (RTM)[6] (see figure 5.4).

In the early days of developing cranial osteopathy, Dr. Sutherland observed that tension in either the falx or tentorium would influence the other membrane.[7] For example, when the falx was taut, the tentorium was slack, and vice versa. This is where the concept of reciprocal tension came from. Dr. Sutherland recognized the RTM as one of five essential components of the craniosacral system (figure 7.1). The others are motility of the central nervous system (inner tide), cerebrospinal fluid, mobility of cranial bones, and involuntary sacral motion between the ilia (pelvic bones).[8]

To envision the reciprocal tension membrane in action, imagine a fish tank with hammocks suspended inside, attaching to the front, back, and sides. The hammocks are neither too taut nor too slack, so that whatever is placed inside them (in this case your brain) stays in the very center. The hammocks provide support from above, below, and around the sides, making your brain seem weightless; no matter how the tank is moved, your brain never touches the sides. This is an ideal scenario for your brain, because its cells are so delicate. Should the brain touch your skull, brain damage results. This is in fact the definition of a concussion.

Now let's try an experiment. What happens if one of the hammocks is pulled extra tight? Your brain will no longer rest in the middle of the tank but rather will be forced off to one side—but not quite so much as to actually touch the side of the tank. Depending on which hammock you tighten or loosen, your brain will sink or rise, shift right or left. This is a demonstration of reciprocal tension. This idea becomes more significant when we realize that the membranes inside your head are continuous with the fasciae of your entire body.

Living brain tissue is dynamic and responsive to pressures. If any part of the falx or tentorium is tight, it can impact brain functioning, having repercussions throughout your body. Restrictions in the RTM can influence a wide range of conditions, including obsessive-compulsive disorder (OCD), attention deficit (ADD), and hyperactivity (ADHD), among others. The advancement of brain mapping in the past thirty years has taught us how to locate portions of the brain that address specific functions, which helps cranial practitioners to more specifically address conditions that may be influenced by membranous tension. Of course, a practitioner is primarily following their

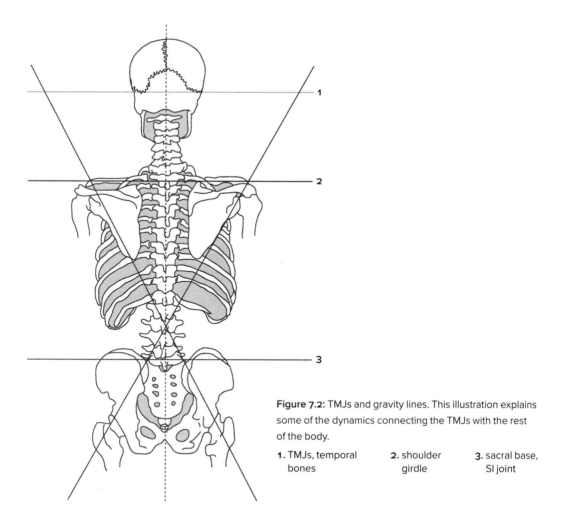

Figure 7.2: TMJs and gravity lines. This illustration explains some of the dynamics connecting the TMJs with the rest of the body.

1. TMJs, temporal bones   **2.** shoulder girdle   **3.** sacral base, SI joint

felt sense of the tissues. But perhaps even more fascinating is the recognition that *you* can release restrictions within the RTM through the way you move your body and focus your mind. Figure 7.2 provides a visual of common cross-connections. Let's explore this viscerally.

Right Body/Left Body

Have you ever noticed that one side of your body tends to be tighter? Take a moment to stand and breathe, feeling your body. Bring attention to your feet contacting the floor, the length of your legs as you stand, your hips, the length of your torso, your shoulders, your arms as they rest at your side, your neck and head. Now start to notice the little or big differences between the right and left sides of your body. Which foot rests more heavily on the floor?

Do you naturally place more weight on one leg? Does one leg feel stronger than the other? What about your hips, are they level? Or is one hip slightly higher? Now perceive your torso. Does it feel straight? Or does it lean a little to one side or the other? And your shoulders, is one higher? What about your arms? Is there one arm you rely on when you have difficulty opening a jar, because you know it's stronger? And your head, is it centered over your body, or does it lean forward or back or to one side?

Now go and stand in front of a mirror. Look with your gentle, subtle vision. Which leg has more muscle tone or seems stronger? Which hip is higher? Placing your hands on the tops of your hips can help to make this more apparent. And which shoulder? This one is usually pretty obvious. Which arm is more toned? What about your neck and head, do they pull slightly to one side? These imbalances are perfectly natural and are in some way a reflection of the membranes inside your head. We'll explore this more through the yoga in part two of this book. An understanding of the RTM is an important aspect of our TMJ yoga program.

Midline—Moshe's Story Continues

You might remember the story of Moshe, the boy who developed a tic after getting braces on his teeth. Years before that tic, when Moshe first came into my office at the age of six, he was expressing attention deficit and hyperactivity (ADHD). His kindergarten teachers were challenged by his apparent inattentiveness and need to constantly move. They were advocating for pharmaceutical regulation of his moods and felt he wasn't ready to go on to the next grade level. They suggested he spend more time in kindergarten— not due to a lack of intelligence but in accordance with their strict behavioral standards.

As I worked with Moshe, a few things stood out. The fasciae were rigid throughout his body, including within his head. It struck me that rigid fasciae must be very uncomfortable. Every time he'd become a little bit quiet and still inside, I'm guessing it would feel like being trapped in something very tight, as if he were wearing a suit that was a few sizes too small. It would be instinctual to move to get away from this feeling. The resulting need to move might well be interpreted as restlessness and inattention.

Fascia is a thin casing of connective tissue that surrounds every bone, muscle, organ, blood vessel, and nerve fiber, giving these structures extra strength and resilience. You might think of it as a layer of Saran Wrap encasing your body parts, supporting order and harmony within. Fascia can be elastic or rigid. It is constantly responding to our environment, how we feel, what we eat, and most importantly, how much we move. Truly, it forms a web of connectivity throughout the body. We might liken it to the irrigation system of Gaia, with its many little springs and wells and seepings of moisture, that connects, liquefies, and offers resilience to our structure.

Take a closer look back at figure 7.2. The RTM is a big player in right-left imbalances in your body. These imbalances exist when we are born and are most often amplified over the course of our lives, corresponding to the complexity of life experience, our brains, how we use our bodies, and the force of gravity constantly bearing down on us.

Returning to Moshe, the rigidity of his fasciae was coupled with the lack of a strong midline. The midline is a central vertical axis around which information is organized, and it's an important concept in many healing modalities. In Chinese medicine this central axis is called the governor and conception vessels. In Ayurveda and yoga, it's the sushumna channel. In craniosacral, the midline is considered to have embryological origins[9]: The *primitive streak* is a developmental stage common to reptiles, birds, and mammals. In humans this appears at twenty-one days of development in utero. The streak grows from tail to head, orienting the fetus. It will form the nervous system and provide the foundation for the fetus's further growth and development. The midline is also closely associated with the dural tube. Midline disturbances are often nervous system disturbances that have originated in early childhood or during gestation.

The longer I worked with Moshe, the more I began to wonder about the trauma history of his parents. His symptoms seemed to indicate a significant nervous system disruption, but it did not appear as though anything traumatic had occurred directly to him. I knew his parents to be caring, loving, and highly conscientious. Not that this makes trauma impossible, just less likely. His parents were both born in Afghanistan. They grew up knowing one another, first in their home country and later as a part of the Afghan refugee community in France. I asked Moshe's mother whether the long-standing civil war had begun before she left her childhood home. "Yes, for sure" was her reply. Her family departed for France in 1980 following the Russian invasion. She was thirteen. I suspect Moshe's symptoms were an expression of intergenerational trauma.[10]

Stress and trauma have genetic markers. The field of epigenetics teaches us that genes can be turned on and off in response to a wide range of factors including diet, lifestyle, and our environment. If your parents or grandparents were exposed to violence and trauma that they had no opportunity to heal, this changed their nervous system and your genetic makeup.[11] The egg that became you was developed in your grandmother's womb. Her immediate life experience was transmitted to you through DNA. Those who have been fortunate to not directly experience war may find they are unraveling the unexpressed trauma of their ancestors. This presents us with a tremendous opportunity for healing.

Moshe's weak midline and rigid fascia informed me as to how to help him. In addition to using craniosacral techniques, we did yoga and breath work to remind his body of the experience of fluidity and reawaken his midline. We started with balance poses, which are wonderful for strengthening the midline and present a fun challenge for most children. We also put together a mini-sun salutation sequence made of up Downward Dog, Cobra, and Child's Pose to release his neck and shoulder muscles while also building core strength and suppleness. Adding one new pose every week or two to create the full sequence kept it interesting. Three-Part Breathing (page 212) helped Moshe cultivate self-regulation. He began to realize it was a "portable practice" he could do anywhere, discreetly without anyone knowing, just to help himself feel better. Gradually he became less brittle and reactive and more able to access relaxed and calm states on his own.

Periodically checking in with Moshe's mother, I developed playful tasks for homework the family could do to somatically reinforce what Moshe was learning. After eight weeks we saw significant changes in his capacity for attention and being still. By then, the school year was coming to an end. As they were leaving for summer vacation, Moshe's mom said, as an afterthought, "Oh, by the way, the school says he can go on to the next grade with the rest of his class. They don't need him to start medication anymore. They're happy with his conduct now."

Bunions—Elizabeth's Story

In the early days of my private practice I got a call from Elizabeth, who wanted relief from bunions. She couldn't find any shoes that felt comfortable and was in constant pain when standing—which was an unavoidable part of her nursing job. Her podiatrist recommended surgery, but she was scared of that option. When she first contacted me, I said, "Bunions? I don't know. But I'm willing to try."

During our first session, as I touched Elizabeth's sacrum, I found it was very tight and suspected it was uncomfortable for her. She hadn't mentioned this during intake, though, so I grew curious. Her reply was simply, "Oh yeah, car accidents happened years ago. I haven't been the same since. I started clenching after that." Her tail was happy to receive the attention. After it came into greater balance, I moved on to her head and neck, which were also surprisingly tight. *Hmm . . . Could this possibly be the origin of her foot pain?* The pieces of this mysterious puzzle were starting to come together.

She returned the following week saying, "I went for a walk without pain for the first time in as long as I can remember. It was one of those things where I just went out and did it, and then when I got back realized what I had just done. It felt great!" While I worked with her head and neck in our second session, Elizabeth became deeply relaxed. In this serene state, her head suddenly turned dramatically to the left. Several minutes later, her head turned gently back to center—all without my initiating it. Afterward, Elizabeth commented, "When you turned my head to the left, it surprised me because during PT after my car accidents, that was the tight side. It was always difficult to turn that direction." I stopped her to clarify that I had not turned her head; it had turned of its own accord. It took her a few minutes to accept this possibility. When the body moves involuntarily to release restrictions, it is called *unwinding* and is a beautiful example of the body's intelligence and capacity for healing. When conditions are right, the body is fully capable of releasing long-held tensions on its own—spontaneously and completely. As a cranial practitioner, I support this possibility by creating the conditions for unwinding to happen. The same thing can happen during a yoga class or other movement and bodywork modalities, particularly when there is a focus on deep relaxation and conscious awareness of movement.

Before leaving my office Elizabeth tried turning her head to the left, and sure enough, she had more freedom than she had known in a long time. In addition, over the course of the following week she found that the bunion pain was gone. While it may seem hard to believe, the pain in her feet originated in her neck and jaw. It began as whiplash from Elizabeth's car accidents and eventually migrated down to her roots, causing pain at the base of her big toe. How? The core link transmitted restriction patterns from her upper neck to her hips. The restriction affected the way the femurs rested in Elizabeth's hip sockets, which influenced her standing posture and gait, and ultimately put imbalanced pressure on her feet. We are reminded yet again that the entire body is connected. Elizabeth's story shows us how close the feet and jaw are, despite outside appearances.

We cannot easily separate one aspect of the body from another; imbalances in the jaw can be reflected throughout our systems. Imagine a single drop of water falling on a pond: it will send ripples across the entire surface. Likewise, forces of imbalance can be transmitted vast distances through the liquid membrane system of the body and through restrictions of subtle cranial motility. Craniosacral is not the only modality to recognize how interconnected the body is. In reflexology, your whole body is accessed through the feet. In Chinese medicine, your ears provide an entrée to influence all structures.

Hypermobility—Cassandra's Story

"Can I reschedule my appointment for Friday? My doctor is insisting I go in for an MRI. She's concerned it may have been a stroke. I have face droop on the right side!" After getting the all clear on the MRI from her doctor, Cassandra came in reporting an aura from what she believed was a migraine and intense pain on the right side of her head, down her neck, and along her shoulder and arm. "My arm feels weird," she said. "I don't really know where it is. And my jaw is so sore! I guess I've been clenching." Her MRI had shown her discomfort was not due to a stroke but rather nerves that were aggravated. The face droop was resolving itself as she took some time to rest. After she lay down on my table, I passed my hand over her body about three feet above her, moving slowly from head to toe. Immediately I felt the vigilance of the right side of her head, neck, shoulder, upper ribs, and arm. I understood about her arm.

"It seems like your arm isn't quite sure whether it's still part of your body," I said.

"Yes, that's it!" she replied with a laugh. "Oh dear . . . to be honest, I think this happened when I picked up a rock. I squatted down and wrapped my arms around it, and then as I went to straighten my legs and stand up, I immediately felt something . . . Actually, I had a pretty severe dislocation of this shoulder over twenty years ago. I guess I've reinjured it now." After about thirty minutes on my table, she said, "Oh wow, the right side of my body just landed. I guess maybe I have been more stressed than I realized. School, work, money . . . I'm blaming it on cryptocurrency. I thought I'd do it to earn some extra cash, but you know, it's easy to get obsessed. That stuff never shuts down. It's fluctuating 24/7!" Stress and the fight-or-flight activation cause muscular tension. Left brain activity—bills, schedules, deadlines, even just showing up—cause right-side body tension. When muscles are contracted, we don't fully rest but rather hold ourselves separate, from the floor, the bed, any surface we are touching, from others, and from our environment in general. For sure, this can lead to a sense of disconnection. As Cassandra began to relax, her body could rest more fully. The right side of her body literally dropped onto the table. We might say she was arriving in the present moment.

Elemental/Constitutional View: Wind, Fire, Water, Earth

Cassandra was a dancer, performer, artist, and student—a highly creative individual. She was completing her PhD while running a unique business producing clothing that lights up different colors in response to the emotions of the wearer. Constitutionally, her joints were hypermobile, and she'd had several injuries as a result. She began clenching as a teenager.

Hypermobility is related to the connective tissue or fascia. Ayurveda understands this to be an expression of the *vata* or wind constitution, because of its association with the joints. There are three primary constitutions, based on qualities of the elements: wind (*vata*), fire (*pitta*), and earth and water combined together (*kapha*). Hypermobile individuals face some unique challenges in life. While it may look appealing to be so flexible—especially if you're into yoga—if you're hypermobile you actually need to learn to stretch in a different way. Because your joints are loose, it initially seems like you can perform yoga poses more easily than many people. Stretching the joints feels really good too—endorphins are released, and it can have an addictive quality. However, when the joints are regularly overstretched, they become weaker and less stable. Additionally, your muscles underwork when your joints overwork. That means your muscles can stay relatively weak and contracted even when you appear to be performing some fabulous stretches. A hypermobile individual is tasked with retraining the way they stretch—

paying close attention to stabilizing their joints and bringing the stretch into the belly of their muscles. It is an important process to learn how to not overstretch the ligaments, tendons, or joints. We can all benefit from paying attention to the challenges faced by hypermobile individuals. Because no one has a perfectly balanced body, each one of us expresses some amount of imbalanced right-left patterning. Aging tends to increase this, as well as to make joints more vulnerable. Thus we all experience some form of the complex dynamics involved in hypermobility.

There is an interesting relationship between hypermobility and TMD. The ligaments that guide the disc that sits in the TMJs can become overstretched through clenching, causing lots of popping, clicking, and grinding. It becomes more important to not overstretch your jaw when opening your mouth, as you may be more prone to dislocation. Additionally, recognizing—and minimizing—right-left imbalances is very important. For Cassandra, her left side tended to be the stabilizing side, and her right side was more prone to "giving" when under duress. Hence her right shoulder gave when the rock was just too heavy to lift. Being under stress didn't help. The more her left brain got preoccupied with the many details of her life—schedules, money, homework, business, and so on—the more the muscles on her right side contracted, which made her joints become increasingly vulnerable to overstretching.

Yin and Yang

Right-left imbalances originate in brain activity, which in turn influences the reciprocal tension membrane. Imbalances are then transmitted through the dura to the fascia throughout your body. What this means is, how you use your brain—what tasks you are asking it to perform—influences your relative state of balance. This is revealed in your physical structure: the right and left sides of your body. The right hemisphere controls the left side of your body; the left hemisphere corresponds to the right side of your body. While the brain is complex, we do have some simple correlations with right and left hemisphere activity. Left brain (right body) is associated with the rational mind and linear thinking—for example, money, schedules, showing up on time, and completing tasks. Energetically the right side embodies the *yang* or masculine qualities of action, strength, focus, hardness, and quickness. Elementally it is associated with the sun, fire, and heat. The sun also refers to daytime, the aspects that shine brightly in our worldly endeavors. Your right brain corresponds to the left side of your body and is associated with *yin* qualities of softness, receptivity, and intuition. This represents the feminine or lunar aspect of our being, including darkness, nighttime, and going inward for meditation and contemplation.

It's important to recognize we each have both feminine and masculine—yin and yang—aspects to our persona. You have your own unique balance of these qualities. However, losing harmony externally makes us vulnerable to disharmony internally—often resulting in injury, stress, trauma, and illness. When we lose our balance in response to the demands of our work life, our personal life, or even a natural disaster or other event that is beyond our control, we can view it as a useful reflection for coming back to center. We might ask ourselves, "Where did I lose my way? What have I begun to focus too much time and energy on, and what have I forgotten that is important to me?"

Thus far we've been taking a journey through some of the causes and repercussions of jaw tension throughout your body, at times dissecting the body into small pieces—but ultimately, we come back to the recognition that our bodies function as a whole unit. Our analytical minds like to parse out different aspects, but this approach shows itself to be insufficient. Separating out pieces may occasionally be helpful, but it will never represent our whole story. It simply cannot encompass the totality of who you are. Looking deeper, we can recognize the unit of one human is interconnected with everyone and everything. Can you fully separate yourself from your family, your community, your life experiences, or the planet Gaia?

The Vietnamese Buddhist monk Thich Nhat Hanh coined a term, *interbeing*, that speaks to our reality of being both autonomous and dependent, both separate and a part of everything. No one part of your body can be separated from any other part. Your jaw is connected to your feet, your sacrum, your heart, your brain, and every other aspect of who you believe yourself to be. The rest of this book focuses on cultivating a direct experience with this interconnectedness through practices that can provide relief from jaw tension. Chapter 8 begins our journey of self-care with an introduction to facial self-massage to both alleviate discomfort and help you learn more about your personal tension patterns. Additionally, we'll explore conscious touch, inviting you to experience your body in a new way. Parts two and three of this book offer a wide range of self-help techniques, including core actions for postural alignment, yoga poses, breathing practices, mindfulness, and loving-kindness. I hope you will enjoy the investigation into ways of helping yourself. May these practices be a support to you on your journey to heal jaw tension and come into a sense of wholeness of being.

8

Conscious Healing Touch and Facial Self-Massage for TMD

THERE ARE MANY ways to touch and be touched. In the United States, physical touch is often less common than many places around the globe. A classic study conducted in 1966 observed how many times people touched in cafés around the world. The results were dramatic—London: 0, Florida: 2, Paris: 110, Puerto Rico: 180. In 1999 professor and touch researcher Tiffany Field updated this study, observing teenagers in McDonald's restaurants in Miami and Paris. The results were similar.[1] Terms like *skin hunger*,[2] *touch starved*, and *touch deprivation*[3] became symbolic of the 2020 pandemic when the simplest of contact was deemed unsafe due to novel coronavirus. The painful repercussions of lack of touch, alongside recognition of the many benefits of touch, were finally discussed in newspapers, journals, and our culture at large. Evidence shows touch can decrease stress and cortisol levels; lower blood pressure and heart rate; calm your nervous system; boost dopamine (which decreases depression and increases motivation), serotonin (supporting positive moods and feelings of well-being), and oxytocin (bonding hormone); decrease pain; and improve healing from injuries.[4] All that comes from a little touch. Indeed, touch has the potential to nourish and restore, soothe and repair not only the tissues of your body but also your mind. Touch can improve your sense of well-being and your connection to yourself and to others.

Early in life, touch is essential for healthy brain development. A terrible example of the detrimental effects of lack of touch came to light in 1990 as the existence of Romanian "child gulags" was revealed to the world.[5] Under the communist dictator Nicolae Ceaușescu procreation was encouraged, birth control was unavailable, and poverty was devastating. These policies resulted in many children being left at orphanages where they were severely deprived—loss of touch being central to their situation. Thirty years later the aftereffect is a generation of folx who have tremendous difficulty bonding with others, feeling at ease, or enjoying life.[6] These painful insights have contributed to important changes in our care of children and infants. Thanks to the research of Dr. Field and others, we know that skin-to-skin contact for babies is extremely beneficial—we might even say essential. For preemies it can be lifesaving. Preterm infants who spend "kangaroo time" resting on their parents' bodies have normal brain development by adolescence, as contrasted to those who remain in incubators.[7]

Conscious Touch

We have seen in some of the client stories in the previous chapters that unconscious touch can cause trauma. If there is an intent to harm, control, or manipulate, this will be transmitted through our touch. When we touch with aggression or from a place of personal need, this can negatively impact the person we are touching. We are sensitive beings. Mood, emotion, feeling, desire, and intention can all be conveyed through touch.

It turns out that different qualities of touch influence different nerves. Quick touch travels along big, insulated (myelinated) nerve fibers.[8] We can think of these as busy freeways where the drivers are mostly focused on getting somewhere quickly. Slow touch, however, travels on small unmyelinated nerve fibers. We might liken these to meandering country roads, where we can focus more on the journey. Unfortunately, a lot of massage and bodywork focuses on deep, heavy pressure with an intent to manipulate and change your body. Let's unlearn that approach. Instead, I want to invite you to take your time. How would it be to touch with the intention to listen from within? Let go of the desire to fix or repair. Just be present with whatever shows up under your hands. Stay in the present moment. There's nothing to do and nowhere to go. Allow yourself to enjoy the ride. Dr. Sutherland coined the phrase *with thinking fingers*, meaning to touch with intelligence, presence, and a sincere interest in listening to the wisdom of the organism you are touching. Listening in this case is an inward activity, done through your hands and body rather than your ears.

Self-Touch Experiment

Here's an experiment in cultivating mindful touch. Place your hand on your thigh. Notice what is under your hand. It's OK to close your eyes, particularly if that helps you to connect with your inner experience. Become receptive. What is here? Does your thigh feel warm or cool? Hard or soft? Let your hand rest lightly, without trying to do anything.

As you keep your hand on your thigh, you may begin to notice tingling, pulsation, or other sensations under your hand. See if you can differentiate the different layers of tissues under your hand. First, there is skin. Skin usually has a pliable quality. Next there is fascia, which most often feels fluid. Then there is muscle, which can be hard or soft or in between. And then at the center there is bone, which is dense, solid. Play with the possibility of moving your awareness between these different layers of your body.

Now see whether you can expand your awareness to perceive your thigh as connected to the rest of your body. Keeping your hand still, with a light quality of touch that feels *almost* (but not quite) as though it were hovering above your leg, feel how your thigh connects to your knee, lower leg, and foot. And then notice the connection between your thigh, your hips, and your torso. Let your awareness travel through your body from your hand contact—not simply from your imagination but rather from the tactile sense of cells connecting to cells to form a body that is yours.

It's fine to open your eyes at any time. This can be helpful if you space out or feel confused. Take a few mindful breaths, noticing your belly expanding and releasing and how your body is oriented in space. Feel the places your body touches—the chair, sofa, or floor.

Shared Touch Experiment

Now let's experiment with touching someone else. Ask a friend to try this with you. Place your hand on their arm. As above, notice your experience. Become curious. Is their arm cool or warm? Let your hand rest lightly. Can you feel movement under your hand? Pulsation, throbbing, or perhaps little tugs in different directions?

Now try to perceive the different layers of tissues. Notice the elastic quality of skin. And then sense the resilient fluid quality of membrane (fascia). Below this is muscle. Muscles are highly changeable—they become suppler when they are warmed up, more rigid or denser when they are unused, flaccid when they are weak, solid when they are strong. What qualities are apparent right now? Below muscle is bone. If you are touching your friend's forearm, then there are two bones: the radius and ulna. See whether you can perceive the difference and the space between them, filled with muscles, tendons, ligaments, fluid, and fascia.

Now try to perceive their arm as connected to the rest of their body. Let your awareness expand through your tactile sense of contact. In one direction lies their wrist, hand, and fingers. In the other direction lies their upper arm, shoulder, and torso. Experiment with perceiving their entire body through this one contact while keeping your quality of touch very light.

When you are ready to end, sit quietly for a moment, noticing your breathing. How does your body feel now? Have things changed within your own body as a result of touching someone else consciously? When you are ready, talk with your friend about their experience. Take time to simply listen before sharing your own experience.

TMD Facial Massage

The massage sequence presented below can help you in several ways. The most straightforward benefit is immediate relief. Touching your own face and jaw consciously can allow your muscles to relax, which can decrease pain and discomfort. It's that simple. It can also help you to stop clenching right away. The quicker you stop clenching, the faster you stop causing harm to yourself.

Frequent self-massage will also help you to track your tension patterns. Practicing this sequence several times a day, every day, will allow you to notice what time of day your jaw tends to be tighter (Is it first thing in the morning? Or at the end of the day?) and when it is looser. We might call this *building a library of experience* regarding your jaw tension. Keep notes about this in your journal. In addition to noticing your regular patterns, over time you will observe irregularities. This includes times when your jaw is unusually tight or especially relaxed. This is also extremely helpful information. The recognition of changes in your relative level of jaw tension invites reflection regarding what has changed in your life. Did you just come out of a meeting with your boss? Are you returning from vacation? Was there a family crisis? Is it related to your hormonal cycle?

Knowledge is power. The closer you track your jaw tension, the likelier you will be able to observe cause and effect. Learning what causes tension gives you the opportunity to make wise choices. Is there something you can reduce or avoid doing in your life—for example, chewing gum? If the source of tension is unavoidable—meetings with your boss comes to mind—then you are empowered to work mindfully with the situation, perhaps by offering loving-kindness to yourself *and* your boss before the meeting. Doing some gentle body movement or mindful breathing may also be of benefit. It is entirely possible to change your relationship to the stressful situations that cause you to clench.

Frequent self-massage is an excellent form of biofeedback. With a listening quality of touch you will learn to feel when your muscles are tight and when they are relaxed. It becomes an empowering tool for self-awareness and care—one you can have fun with!

Step-by-Step Approach

The massage techniques below are best practiced while sitting with the back of your head resting against something or while lying down. Keep your mouth slightly open at all times when massaging; it is important that your upper and lower teeth not be touching. Keeping your mouth slightly open can serve as a reminder, ensuring there is a little space between the upper and lower teeth. If you find your fingers catching on your skin, try putting a little lotion or oil on your fingertips for a bit more glide.

Try doing this sequence three to five times a day: first thing in the morning, at midday, at night before going to bed, and a couple other quiet moments as they fit into your routine. Of course, if you only get to it once a day, that's alright too. This ten-step massage sequence will probably take around fifteen minutes to complete, although you are welcome to take longer. If you're pressed for time, you can skip the first four steps—just do steps five through ten. This shorter sequence takes about five minutes but can still release tension in your TMJs.

Different muscles prefer different qualities of touch. For example, the masseter is the strongest muscle in your body, with big bunchy muscle fibers. It often likes a deeper pressure. Temporalis, on the other hand, is a flatter muscle covering several bones (figure 2.8a). It may need a lighter touch. Cheekbones (zygomata) don't like to be compressed but rather enjoy being lifted up (think face-lift), so it's nice to get up under them. And brows love to be spread and unfurrowed. Craniosacral practitioners most commonly use about five grams of pressure, or the weight of a nickel. Try starting with a light touch. Over several minutes you can gradually increase pressure until it feels just right for you, today. Listen to your body, and try to avoid accomplishing a task—for example, trying to get rid of something. You are allowed to just enjoy touching yourself.

Facial Self-Massage Instructions

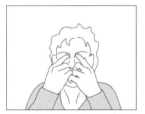

Figure 8.1: Browline pressure point.

1. **Brow Line Pressure Point:** Place the tips of your thumbs at the inner corners of your brow line. Feel for the tender spot. Press up toward the crown of your head, and drag the thumbs slightly away from one another (figure 8.1).

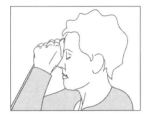

Figure 8.2: Forehead sweep—side view.

2. **Brow Sweep:** Continue to drag the thumb tips away from each other along the brow line to the end of your eyebrows.

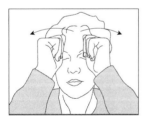

Figure 8.3: Forehead sweep—front view. Arrows indicate the direction of the sweeping motion.

3. **Forehead Sweep:** Place the lower portion of your thumbs side by side on your forehead. Drag your thumbs slightly up toward the crown of your head to traction your skin (figures 8.2, 8.3).

4. **Temples:** Sweep your thumbs away from each other, across your forehead, to the outer edges of your eyebrows, ending at your temples (figure 8.4).

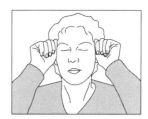

Figure 8.4: Temples—front view.

(For a shorter sequence, start here.)

5. **Masseter Release—Fingertips:** Bring the pads of your three middle fingers to the upper edge of your mandible (lower jaw), just below the ear. Allow your touch to sink in, through the muscle fibers. Then drag down slightly, away from the ears. Feel for tender places (figure 8.5).

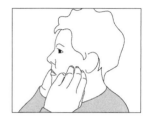

Figure 8.5: Masseter release with fingers.

6. **Masseter Sweep—Knuckles:** Bring the knuckles of your three middle fingers to the upper edge of your mandible (lower jaw), just below the ears (figure 8.6). Allow your touch to sink in, through the muscle fibers. Feel for tender places (figure 8.7).

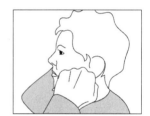

Figure 8.6: Masseter release with knuckles.

7. **Lateral Pterygoid:** Allow your mouth to open, and let the lower jaw hang down as you stroke downward and away from your ears with your knuckles. (Note: you will not be able to access the lateral pterygoid with your mouth closed due to its position.)

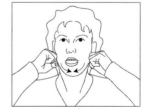

Figure 8.7: Masseter sweep. Arrows indicate the direction of the sweeping motion.

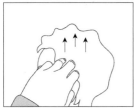

Figure 8.8: Temporalis release. Arrows indicate the direction of the *intention* for release.

8. **Temporalis Release:** Place the fingertips of your middle three fingers on the sides of your head, about one inch above the ears, behind the hairline (figure 8.8). Allow your touch to sink in, and then traction up toward the crown of your head. Note: it's especially nice if you can get a friend to do this on you.

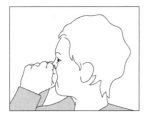

Figure 8.9: Cheekbone pressure point.

9. **Cheekbone Pressure Point:** Place the upper portion of your thumbs onto your cheekbones just below and beside the nose, so that the middle knuckle is under the cheekbone (figure 8.9).

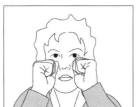

Figure 8.10: Cheekbone sweep—start.

10. **Cheekbone Sweep:** Gently sweep the thumbs away from each other, lifting and supporting the cheekbones, ending at the outer edges of the cheekbones, near the ears (figures 8.10, 8.11).

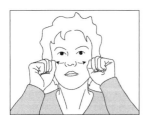

Figure 8.11: Cheekbone sweep—end. Arrows indicate the direction of the sweeping motion.

PART TWO
Yoga for Relief

9

Getting Started

FROM HERE ON, this book details self-help techniques you can put into action to support recovery from jaw tension. The yoga practices in part two and mindfulness exercises in part three are based on practices that have helped thousands of clients and students over the past twenty years; however, they are also rooted in much older traditions. There are places where these disciplines are similar, and areas where they differ. For our purposes, the yoga postures and breathing exercises we are exploring are a collection of physical practices that bring mind and body together, with the potential for a depth of integration and healing. Mindfulness is the quality of attention we bring to our daily lives that allows for recognition of experience, as well as a more continuous awareness. Likewise, this is a healing quality of mind with benefits for your whole being. The principle of ehipassiko—trusting one's deepest experience—is very important to keep in mind. As you explore the practices presented here, please maintain a reflective approach. Notice what you enjoy, what challenges you, and what seems to help. Building confidence in your experience is a form of healing in and of itself.

How Can Yoga and Mindfulness Help?

There are a variety of ways in which yoga has the potential to bring relief. One is quite simply stress reduction. A regular yoga practice has been demonstrated to be an excellent way of changing our relationship to life's challenges and taking care of our body, mind, and heart. This is backed up by extensive research conducted over many years.[1] Similarly, mindfulness has proven health benefits,[2] not the least of which include decreasing anxiety, increasing calm, impulse control, and overall sense of well-being. Mindfulness also supports greater self-awareness, which is very helpful in our journey to reduce jaw tension.

Yoga and mindfulness teach us to observe our body as well as our mind. For example, we can begin to observe our emotional responses and reactions. With regular practice we can notice habit patterns and may see where they come from, how they started, and what the results are when we act out of them. This gives us the opportunity to choose how we respond to people or situations.

You may also learn to feel the direct connection within your body to what is going on around you. For example, how does it feel when you are criticized? Does something tighten in your mind? Can you feel it in your body? Where does it land for you in your being? What about when you are praised—how does that feel in your mind? What about in your body—perhaps something softens?

Developing a yoga practice is very empowering. It teaches us that we can make a difference in our lives. By taking a little time each day to move ourselves through yoga poses, breath awareness, and meditation practices, we see things change in our body and mind. Over time, this becomes like a personal apothecary, your very own storehouse of healing remedies that you can apply with intelligence and wisdom for greater ease and well-being. Once developed, no one can ever take this information away from you. It is your personal treasure trove.

Yoga is fun, easy, and low cost! It is such a delightful, joyous, and beautiful way to engage with ourselves and others. Why not do it?

Developing a Yoga Program for Jaw Tension

The yoga program provided here is informed by the understanding that we can help the jaw to release by working with other parts of the body. The illustration of TMJs and horizontal gravity lines provides a road map for how we will work (see figure 7.2). First let's take a look at the horizontal lines. These demonstrate important points of influence between the TMJs and the rest of the body. The shoulders and pelvis are key areas for our yoga practice to focus on building greater awareness and proper alignment. We will also include the feet because they are the foundation upon which we stand. Your feet are your roots, your connection to Mother Earth.

Now let's look at the diagonal lines. These demonstrate the impact of gravity when there are structural imbalances. No one has a perfectly balanced body. Everyone has a perfectly imbalanced body. This is a beautiful expression of our humanity. One leg is just a little shorter than the other, one hip a little higher, one shoulder a little rotated. Gravity is a constant force pressing down on us and having a continual impact that we cannot escape. The force of gravity can be transmitted on a diagonal particularly where the imbalances are greater.

On a practical level this means your aches, pains, and structural imbalances may not be all on one side of your body. They may carve a diagonal line or a zigzag. For example, is it your right TMJ, left shoulder, right hip, and left foot that tend to bother you? Or is it your left jaw and shoulder and right hip and foot? Over the course of this yoga program, you can begin to develop a clearer sense of how things stack up in your body. The benefit to this understanding is this: When we know how things stack up, we can learn how to unstack them, which means a greater understanding of cause and effect, and ultimately the potential for less pain and more freedom of body, mind, and heart.

The diagonal lines highlight the TMJs, shoulder blades, sacroiliac joints, and heads of the thighbones where they rest in the hip sockets. This gives us a little more precision with regard to where to focus in our yoga practice.

We'll start our yoga program with a few foundational practices called *core actions*, which are designed to access specific structural awareness in the hips, shoulders, and jaw. Then we'll apply these to specific yoga poses. Since the goal is to relieve jaw tension, it is important to keep returning to an awareness of your mouth and jaw in every pose. Please read the instructions for each pose carefully before proceeding to the yoga sequence section. I encourage beginners and experienced yoga practitioners alike to go step by step with implementing this program. If you have practiced yoga before, it will still be very helpful for you to learn how to practice yoga to relieve jaw tension as described in this program. Some aspects of this approach may be unfamiliar even to longtime yogis.

Action vs. Movement

The best and most beautiful things in the world cannot be seen or even touched. They must be felt with the heart.

—HELEN KELLER

Our yoga program begins with a series of core actions that lay a foundation for how we practice to relieve jaw tension. These actions will inform the yoga poses that follow. The core actions can also be practiced independently of yoga poses to inform your posture and body movements in daily life. In order to better understand this, let's look closely at what distinguishes *actions* from *movements*.

With a movement, the physical body changes position in some demonstrable way. Examples include raising your arm, lifting your leg, or bending over and placing your hands on the floor.

With an action, the physical movement is very small. For example, you might rotate your thighbone, connect your shoulder blades to your ribs, or lift your upper sternum. You won't see much—if any—external change if you look with your normal vision. However, with actions there is an intention to affect your body's alignment in a way that is beneficial. Actions focus on very specific, often minute portions of the body. They hone your awareness, refining your capacity to work skillfully. Actions are intended to bring greater harmony, improving overall alignment and well-being.

Actions are a bridge between body and mind. They are an important piece of what makes yoga more than just a physical practice. Action instructions can seem impossible. I mean, who can "rotate the femur head"—and what does that mean anyway? How will the shoulder blades ever connect with the ribs? How can we know when we get it right?! Actions bring relief. It just feels good when you get it right. It is somehow satisfying within the body. If we look with our inner eye—*if we feel while we see*—we will notice a distinct change when the action is performed.

Actions require a refinement of effort. Sometimes we work very hard, and our effort gets in the way. Try softening your breath, relaxing a bit, and focusing gently on your body. *Relaxing* does not mean that we don't try or that our body gets all soft and floppy. Rather, in this context it means doing more with less stress, accessing the action through ease rather than struggle. In this sense, actions teach us to use the mind wisely so that it becomes a friend in our yoga practice and our lives. This lesson can be applied anywhere in life.

It's important to notice the breath as we practice. Anything that helps the breath to soften, relax, and grow deeper and smoother is moving in the right direction. While deepening a pose may shorten the breath or briefly cause a disturbance, we should be able to bring balance back to the breath within a few seconds. If not, it's wise to back off. When performing an action, let the breath be your guide. Is the breath becoming gentler, easier, more refined? This is a good direction.

What about your mind? How does it feel, what qualities are present? Performing an action might cause some momentary agitation, but again, we should be able to stabilize things within a few breaths. Ultimately the action should result in a peaceful and joyous mind state, or *sukha* (the Sanskrit word for spiritual contentment). Sukha means we are happy and contented with what is. This is a happiness that does not require getting what we want or anyone else to change. Sukha connotes being without struggle, deeply at ease. Actions result in sukha.

If you are already familiar with yoga postures, please practice the core actions anyway before moving on to the poses and sequences in this book. This will help you to better understand our approach. Once you are familiar with the core actions, progress to the yoga poses. Please also take the time to carefully read the yoga pose instructions, as it may be different from what you have experienced elsewhere. This is a specialized program with unique applications. The core actions will be integrated into each yoga posture. From there you can find the yoga sequence that best matches your ability.

For people who are less familiar with yoga, the core actions are a great way to begin working with your body to bring relief from jaw tension. These actions can be practiced anywhere, anytime, without any props or special environments. Truth be told, I practice these core actions every day, many times a day. I find them beneficial even when my personal practice is not particularly related to relieving jaw tension.

The core actions presented here will support greater self-awareness and overall postural well-being. Try applying them while standing in line at the grocery store (jaw, shoulders, hips, and feet), first thing in the morning upon standing up (hips and jaw), or when first sitting down in your car seat (hips, shoulders, jaw). If you work a desk job, stand up at least once every hour and take a minute or two to apply all four core actions. Notice how you feel before and after. Odds are good it will be refreshing to both your body and mind to take a little inner break in this way.

Mapping Your Personal Tension Pattern

As you go through the exercises in the following chapters, you will develop a deeper understanding of how your body holds tension and what causes your patterns of pain. In the Mapping Your Body exercise, we will map your personal tension pattern. Please take this exercise lightly and enjoy the process. Have fun with it!

It's important to recognize that pain does not necessarily mean muscles are chronically tight. Pain can also be a sign that your muscles are being overstretched or that you have loose joints. So how do we know what is tight and what is loose? Range of motion can be a good indicator. For example: Which side of your mouth opens more widely? Which shoulder has greater range of motion? Which hip allows you to go more deeply into a yoga pose? These are the looser sides. The side with less range of motion is the tight side.

Our bodies often have a side that tends to be more stable and a side that tends to be more willing to "give" or compensate. The stabilizing side is often stronger and tends to carry more tension in the muscles. When we are under stress, the stabilizing side may contract more . . . and more . . . eventually causing the "giving" side to overstretch. If this pattern continues, at some point the stabilizing side may get so tight that muscles spasm. Then we are inclined to say something like, "My back went out." Meanwhile, on the "giving" side, things are getting stretched beyond their capacity for stability. We may not feel this happening for a long time. This stretching will most often happen in the ligaments or muscle attachments, and it can lead to unstable joints. People with a tendency toward hypermobility are more vulnerable to this. From the Ayurvedic perspective, hypermobility is a constitutional factor (see chapter 7). This means that some people are naturally more prone to this than others.

It is interesting to note that the parts of the body that complain most loudly are often not the cause of the problem. Sometimes we need to look across the aisle to find the true origin of the pain. For example, if your right hip is chronically tight, it may not hurt but may begin to pull on the right or left knee, hip, and even ribs. Instead of continually trying to fix the painful (and overstretched) side, it can be very helpful to realize what *isn't* opening.

With close investigation we can realize the stubborn right hip is the place to work. As we focus in and begin to invite the right hip to open up, miraculously the complaints on the left side of the body may disappear. The entire body is interconnected. We can't really separate one structure from another.

Grow curious about your own body patterns. Trust your experience. Pay attention. Take notes. Start a moon journal where you write down your experiences from your practice and your daily life. Are all your aches/pains/injuries on one side, or do they cross your body—or perhaps form a zig-zag line? Expand your awareness to notice what the patterns of tension are throughout your body. Begin to build a map of experience. In time this will inform your patterns of tension and injury. Try not to rush to conclusions; rather, build a library by taking notes daily. Over time your patterns will become clear. Somewhat like looking at an Escher drawing, the image will change before your very eyes, revealing a beautiful web of interconnection between mind, body, and heart.

EXERCISE: MAPPING YOUR BODY

Props needed: One or two sheets of paper, several colored pens or pencils, a mirror and/or a friend and a cell phone camera

Fold an 8½-by-11-inch sheet of paper in half lengthwise to create a crease. Unfold the paper and write "front" in the upper corner on one side and "back" in the upper corner on the other side. On the back side, add the words "right" in the upper corner on the right side and "left" in the upper corner of the left side of the paper. On the front side, your drawing will be a mirror image, as if it were a photograph of your body. Therefore you will write "left" on the upper right corner and "right" on the upper left corner. When you look at the front of your image, it will be important to remember that right is left and left is right. For this reason, I encourage you to begin drawing on the back side first.

The crease at the center represents your spine. With a pencil, lightly draw a stick figure on the "front" side of the paper using the crease for your spine. Add perpendicular lines representing your shoulder girdle and pelvis, a circle for your head (don't forget your neck), and parallel lines for your arms and legs, which extend from the end of the perpendicular (shoulder and hip) lines. The side marked "front" represents the front of your body. The side marked "back" represents the back of your body.

▪ STEP ONE: DRAWING YOUR BODY

The simplest way to approach this is to have a friend take photos of you from the back and the front. For the photos, stand naturally in a relaxed version of Tadasana, arms at your sides. Don't work too hard to correct all your imbalances; for this project it will be helpful to see your uncorrected posture. It can also be helpful to place your fingertips at the top of your hips in one of the photos. This will help to easily identify any differences between right and left sides.

Looking at the photo of the back of your body, which shoulder is higher? Beginning on the side labeled "back," draw a new line to represent how your shoulders appear, with either the right or left side higher. Which hip bone is higher? Draw a new line to represent how your hips appear, with either the right or left side higher. Is your head centered, or does it tend to fall toward the right or left side? Draw a new circle to represent your head as it appears, tilting to either the right or left side. With your arms at your sides, notice where your hands are relative to your torso, hips, and legs. Does one hand end up lower than the other? Draw arms on the stick figure with your hands ending at the appropriate spot relative to the rest of your body. Notice your feet. Does one foot turn out or in? Draw the legs and feet on your stick figure to represent your normal posture.

Now turn over the paper to trace the lines for your shoulders, hips, arms, legs, and head on the side labeled "front." You may want to stand in front of a mirror in Tadasana so that you can see for yourself which way your head tilts, which shoulder and hip are higher, and which foot turns out or in.

The last piece to drawing your stick figure is your spine. For this you will need someone to observe your bare back. Choosing a person you trust, create a safe environment for this portion of the exercise. If there are sideways curves to your spine, this is an indication of scoliosis. (It's estimated between 2 and 25 percent of people have some degree of scoliosis[3]). You might ask a friend or loved one to take a picture of your spine so that you can see it yourself. It can be very helpful for them to trace the line of your spine with their finger. To do this, stand quietly in Tadasana with your attention focused inward. It's most helpful if they just use one finger to gently follow the line of your vertebrae, going from the back of your head down your neck and back to your hips. Once you have a clear sense of your spine, draw it on the back side of your paper, using the crease as a guide. If your spine is straight, you can simply draw a line along the crease. If there are curves, create a zig-zag line that is true to your spine. Now turn your paper back to the front and trace the line of your spine on this side.

The final step is to add your face. Stand close enough to the mirror to see your whole face, and notice which eye is higher, which cheekbone, ear, and side of your mouth are higher. To minimize distortions, it's best to use a mirror firmly attached to the wall for this exercise.

Now open and close your mouth, looking carefully at the corners where upper and lower lips meet. Which side of your mouth opens wider? Mark this on your drawing. Next look at the midline of your lips. As you open your mouth, which direction does the midline pull toward? You will notice this most distinctly by observing your lower lip. The middle point of your lip will no longer be at the center; it will migrate toward either the right or the left. Mark this on your map. (Note this exercise is included in more detail in the Mirror Exercise on page 207. It is also available as an audio recording.)

Once you have completed this step, just take a moment to observe what you have drawn. This is a representation of your body structure as it is right now. Breathe in and out. Soften to this image.

STEP TWO: ADDING YOUR PAIN AND TENSION PATTERNS

Choose a color to represent the pain you experience. Draw a star at the places where you frequently feel the most pain in your body, then draw a line connecting these points. Are they all on one side of your body (for example: right jaw, right shoulder, right hip, right knee)? Do they cross your body (right jaw, right shoulder, left hip, left knee)? Or do they form a zig-zag pattern (right jaw, left shoulder, right hip, left knee)? Be completely honest—this is your body map, your personal pattern of discomfort. There is no right or wrong here.

Choose a different color to represent the joints where you have greatest range of motion. Draw a small circle to symbolize the more open joints. This means you need to choose one side of your mouth, neck, shoulder, hips, and knees. If you don't know, leave this blank until you have done the yoga portion of this program. The core actions in chapter 10 will help you start to identify which hip and shoulder tend to be tighter. As you work your way through the yoga poses in chapter 11 and the practice sequences in chapter 12, you will gain more information about your body tension patterns.

The side you did not choose is the tight side. Choose a new color and mark these with a plus sign. Notice whether the pain occurs at places that are tight or loose. This is extremely helpful information for working with jaw tension and balancing your body. If the painful side is the loose side, then you need to take care not to overstretch it further. This means learning to stabilize the talkative achy side. Additionally, learning to become more aware of the quiet, stabilizing side that is actually overly tight will be important and beneficial.

If the painful side is also the tight side, then stretching will likely be very helpful. Go slow initially . . . don't get upset if you can't do it all right away. You are learning a new way of being. Please be gentle with yourself. Kindness and patience have tremendous rewards.

Developing a Moon Journal—*For All Genders*

When working with jaw tension it's helpful to create a journal. There are several intentions behind this practice. Writing down your daily symptoms gives you a record to turn to. This way you can know for sure what you are experiencing and how frequently it happens. Through this personal almanac you can observe whether symptoms are increasing or decreasing over time. Recording other important factors like your diet, schedule changes, significant life events, and even unusual weather or natural disasters can help determine what factors might be influencing your jaw tension. If you decide to apply specific interventions, like getting a night guard, trying headache medication, or a new daily routine, the diary can reveal whether these help or harm, often within a few weeks.

As you begin to adopt some of the lifestyle changes recommended here, it can be helpful to record them. Writing down what yoga sequences you do, how much time you spend meditating, and which practices you try will not only support your practice but also give you feedback in short order regarding what you find beneficial. Taking just a few minutes to write about your emotional and bodily experience daily is a proven method of stress reduction and enhancing well-being.[4]

I particularly encourage keeping a moon journal: linking your note taking to the lunar calendar. While women have done this for centuries, I feel this is beneficial for all genders. We are intrinsically connected to—and influenced by—our environment, and yet we like to deny this is so. Somehow, in our modern society, we have tried to convince ourselves of our autonomy from our habitat—to our detriment. A moon calendar invites the reflection of our interbeing. While you have a measure of physical autonomy, your metaphysical nature recognizes your dependence upon, and connection with, everyone and everything. By simply taking a look at the phase of the moon each day as you take a few minutes to write down your experiences, a positive reintegration can take place for all of us.

EXERCISE: CREATING AND MAINTAINING A MOON JOURNAL

Props needed: A journal or notebook

Choose a special notebook to designate as your moon journal. You can design this yourself, find one created by a local artist, or order one of many available online. It can be as simple as a spiral-bound notebook or something more specialized like a cloth hardcover book with blank pages. Lunar calendars are available from a variety of sources (see appendix for references). You might consider taking a little time to turn this into an arts and crafts project, cutting up a lunar calendar and pasting the moon phase images into your chosen paper journal. The embodiment of this task is very grounding and healing in and of itself. Similarly, the physical task of hand writing your entries can be restorative. While I am an advocate of paper journals and hand writing, there are also numerous online versions available, as well as apps for your cell phone.

The following are ideas of what to include in your journal:

- Daily sleep schedule and quality of sleep
- Physical symptoms (aches and pains and where they are in your body, illness, energy level)
- Daily activities including work, days off, vacation, exercise, and mind-body practices
- Diet, weather, emotions, stress level, significant life events, and natural disasters
- For those who are menstruating, include information regarding your cycle— vulation, menses begin and end, quality of flow, and any related symptoms
- If pregnant, include your daily experiences of this journey

Take at least five minutes in the morning and at night to write these down. Taking more time—fifteen to twenty minutes—at least three times a week can be very beneficial and is highly recommended for stress reduction and overall well-being.

☙ 10

Four Core Actions

THE FOUR core actions represent the essential actions underlying the TMD-relief yoga program. To better understand what an action is, check out the "Action vs Movement" section of chapter 9 ("Getting Started," page 112). This focus has come out of years of working with many individuals and seeing what is most commonly affected by jaw tension. Instead of just trying to "fix the jaw," we are taking a whole-body approach. Part one, Jaw Tension Explained, demonstrates how your jaw interconnects with the rest of your body. With the core actions, we are putting this understanding into practice.

Figure 7.2 (page 89) lays a foundation for the core actions (reading chapter 7 will be helpful). The diagonal lines represent the pathway that TMJ imbalances are most likely to follow through your body. This is a result of the combined forces of gravity and body structure. Take particular note of where the horizontal and diagonal lines meet. Accessing these areas of your body with wise intention is our purpose. We'll focus on your jaw, shoulders, hips, and feet. While the feet aren't included in the illustration, any imbalance in your spine or hips will be transmitted down the length of your legs, landing in your feet, and likewise if your feet are out of balance this will be transmitted upward. Your feet are your roots, your earth connection, and thus are both on the receiving end of forces throughout your body and a foundation for your structure as a whole.

The core actions can be practiced independently, and they are also essential to how we perform yoga for relief from jaw tension. Learning to access these actions is fundamental for the full yoga poses offered in the following chapter. As you get to know the core actions, they will inform your personal tension pattern. Refer back to, and update, your body map (described page 115).

Core Action 1: Your Jaw

Mirror Exercise (page 207) and Oral Cavity Guided Meditation (page 210) will support this action.

In our work with jaw tension, we want to consciously undo the habit of clenching. Here's an action that will help: Open your mouth, extend your tongue as far as you can, and exhale. In yoga, this is known as Lion Face Pose

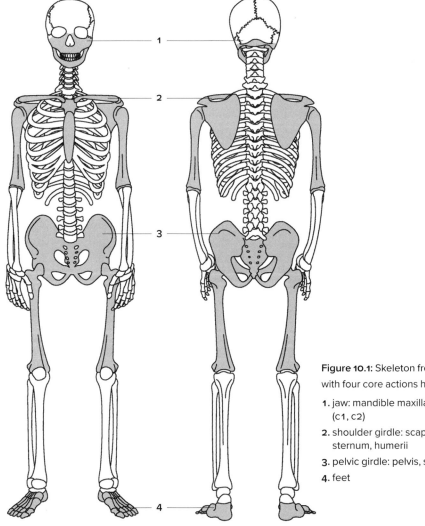

Figure 10.1: Skeleton front and back view with four core actions highlighted.

1. jaw: mandible maxillae, temporals, teeth (c1, c2)

2. shoulder girdle: scapulae, clavicles, sternum, humerii

3. pelvic girdle: pelvis, sacrum, femurs

4. feet

(Simhasana). Imagine a lion roaring its deepest, fiercest roar with a wide-open face. It's impossible to clench while roaring!

When you clench a lot, it can be hard to remember what it is like to *not* clench. Lion Face Pose can function as a reset. When you are intentionally doing something different, you know that you are *not* clenching.

Open your mouth in a way that feels good and provides some amount of release without causing pain. And even more important, *open your mouth with awareness*. Notice what happens to your jaw as you open and close it. Which side opens more easily, right or left? Which side clicks or pops? How do your teeth line up when your mouth is closed—do your upper and lower teeth touch? Try to always keep a little space between the upper and lower teeth, unless of course you are chewing your food. The Mirror Exercise and Oral Cavity Meditation in chapter 15 will help you really notice and better understand your personal tension patterns.

Throughout your day, take a moment here and there to practice your Lion Face Pose. Do it in the bathroom, when you are alone in your office, when you are driving. Be brave: Don't worry what it looks like. Invite your family and friends to do it too! Get to the point where you do this every hour—*and notice what it feels like*. Cultivating an awareness of nonclenching will support you in unraveling the habit of clenching.

We will include Lion Face Pose in many of yoga poses . . . but not all of them. *Do not* do Lion Face Pose when your head is resting against the wall or the floor. When you are lying down on or leaning against a firm surface, there is some chance of the upper neck being jammed by the act of opening your mouth wide—especially when your back is arched. As a result, it is not appropriate to practice Lion Face Pose in conjunction with Bridge Pose (Setu Bandha Sarvangasana) and Reclining Bound Angle Pose (Supta Baddha Konasana): in these poses, keep your mouth closed with teeth apart. (If you have difficulty breathing through your nose, it's fine to open your mouth.) *Do* include Lion Face Pose with all of the standing poses and inverted poses where your head is hanging freely. It will be beneficial in those poses.

The way we practice Lion Face Pose in this program is a little different from how it is often taught. Instead of focusing on maximum range of motion of your jaw and tongue, we will focus more on building awareness regarding how your mouth moves, what feels good, and what is uncomfortable. We're going for quality over quantity. Please read the full instructions before adding it to your yoga program.

Exercise: Lion Face Pose (Simhasana)

Caution: Avoid clicking, popping, or pain in your jaw. If your jaw makes a significant pop when you open it, or if you experience pain, do not open your mouth quite so wide. Find a range of comfort for yourself. How far can you open your mouth without causing it to pop? That's far enough.

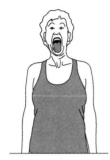

Stand with your feet hip-width apart or sit in any comfortable position. As you exhale, open your mouth wide, extend your tongue, lift your eyebrows, open your eyes wider, and feel your face expand. Breathing in, relax your face and jaw. Allow your mouth to close but keep your upper and lower teeth apart.

Now try it in front of a mirror. Repeat three to five times, and then record your findings on your body map.

Figure 10.2: Lion Face Pose.

Core Action 2: Shoulder Blades

Three-Part Breathing (page 212) and Body Scan Meditation (page 219) will support these actions.

A tight, clenched jaw contributes to a "stress posture" of chronically tight shoulders and a sunken chest. As we learned in part one, there are 136 muscles involved in the movement of your mandible (lower jawbone). That's sixty-eight muscle pairs above and below your jaw—including those involved in shoulder and chest movement. In particular, the trapezius muscle can be chronically contracted and rigid from a combination of over- and underuse. Skillful shoulder work is an important part of our program to relieve jaw tension.

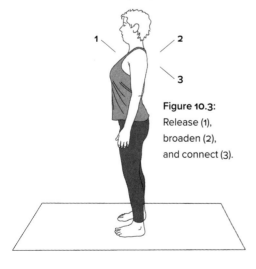

Figure 10.3: Release (1), broaden (2), and connect (3).

The shoulder action is divided into three parts in this program. Through the exercises presented below you will learn to *release*, *broaden*, and *connect* your shoulder blades. It's important to remember that no one part of your body is separate from any other part. Your shoulder blades are connected to the rest of your body. As you work with your shoulders, pay close attention to your chest and upper back. And since our goal is to relieve jaw tension, I encourage you to notice the impact this work has on your head, neck, and jaw posture—as well as how you feel when standing anywhere, anytime.

Shoulder actions can easily be integrated into daily activities—waiting in line at the grocery store, walking down the street, talking on the phone, standing and cooking dinner. My favorite time to practice them is while wearing a backpack. If your pack has a moderate amount of weight in it, it can serve as an excellent reminder to apply the actions described below. We often have a tendency to resist the weight of the pack by lifting our shoulders upward. Experiment instead with *receiving* the weight. Let it teach you to *release, broaden*, and *connect* your shoulder blades. Notice how this allows the pack weight to drop through your skeletal structure, making it easier to support.

The core shoulder actions are applied in yoga poses throughout this program. Each action is progressively subtler, so bring sensitivity and patience to this exploration.

Core Action 2a: Release

EXERCISE: SHRUG

Stand with your arms at your sides. Inhaling, shrug your shoulders up close to your ears (figure 10.4). Exhaling, gently release your shoulder blades down your back and away from your ears as you lift your upper sternum (figure 10.5).

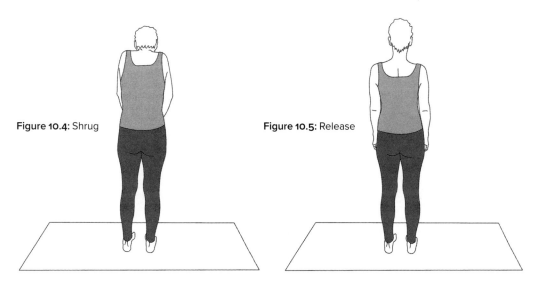

Figure 10.4: Shrug

Figure 10.5: Release

Repeat this three to five times—inhaling, shoulder blades up; exhaling, shoulder blades down and upper sternum lifted.

Keep your mouth relaxed and your upper and lower teeth apart. Add Lion Face Pose on the exhale to be certain you are not clenching.

EXERCISE: REACH AND SHRUG

In this exercise we will repeat the shoulder shrug above, this time with your arms overhead. It's helpful to use a strap around your wrists to keep your arms shoulder-width apart. I'll demonstrate it this way.

Props needed: Yoga strap with buckle (optional)

Stand with your arms at your sides. Place a strap around your wrists, holding your arms shoulder-width apart. Inhaling, reach your arms forward and overhead. Extend through your fingertips with your palms facing each other. Bring your arms in line with your ears, raising your shoulder blades up close to your ears (figure 10.6).

As you exhale, release your shoulders blades down your back and away from your ears as you lift your upper sternum. Keep stretching up through your fingertips with your arms straight overhead. Refrain from arching your back, and be careful that your lower (floating) ribs aren't pushed forward (figure 10.7).

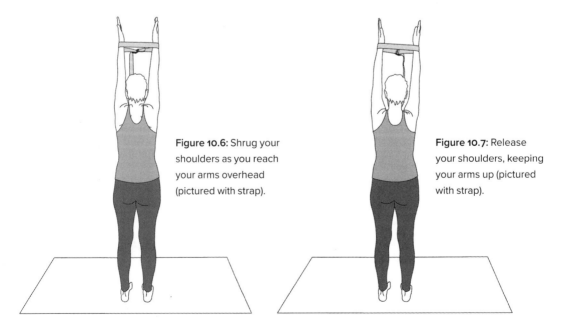

Figure 10.6: Shrug your shoulders as you reach your arms overhead (pictured with strap).

Figure 10.7: Release your shoulders, keeping your arms up (pictured with strap).

Repeat this three to five times: inhaling, stretch your arms and shoulder blades up close to your ears; exhaling, release your shoulder blades down your back while lifting your upper sternum. Keep your mouth relaxed and your upper and lower teeth apart. Add Lion Face Pose on each exhale.

To come out: Exhale as you lower your arms in front of you and down to your sides.

Core Action 2b: Broaden

In the last action, we focused on raising and lowering the shoulder blades. Now the attention shifts to moving your shoulder blades away from one another and broadening your upper back and chest.

Expanding your shoulder blades counteracts the habit of tightening them and activates an underused portion of your trapezius. In addition, it opens your rib cage and frees your breath, inviting relaxation and ease. As we learned in part one, restricted breathing is a common repercussion of jaw tension, with many ill effects.

It's easiest to feel your back and chest broadening when your arms are extended out from your sides at shoulder height. Working at a wall is helpful so that you have something to push into. We'll begin with just one arm at a time.

EXERCISE: SINGLE ARM EXTENDED

Props needed: A wall

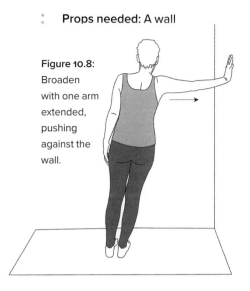

Figure 10.8: Broaden with one arm extended, pushing against the wall.

Stand with the right side of your body near the wall. Place the fingertips of your right hand on the wall at shoulder height with fingers facing up. Then step away from the wall to straighten your arm. Be careful not to hyperextend your elbow.

Now push the wall away while keeping your upper back and chest open and lifted. Notice how your shoulder feels. Add Lion Face Pose as you exhale. Stay for three breaths. (Figure 10.8.)

To come out: Exhale as you release your hand from the wall and let your arm return to your side. Repeat on your other side.

⋮ Exercise: Both Arms Extended in a T

For this action, your shoulder blades—not your arms—lead the movement. Your arms will follow the action initiated by your shoulder blades.

Stand with your feet hip-width apart and arms at your sides. Inhaling, raise your arms overhead as described in the Reach and Shrug exercise above.

On an exhale, lower your shoulder blades down your back and away from each other. Stretch out through your fingertips as you bring your arms down to shoulder height, with your palms facing up and arms parallel to the floor. Balance this stretch through the front and back of your upper body.

With your arms still extended, inhale as you lift your upper sternum and drop your shoulder blades. Exhaling, imagine you are pushing the walls away as you stretch your fingertips in opposite directions allowing your shoulder blades to move away from one another. Feel your upper back and upper chest broaden. Balance the stretch between the upper chest and upper back. (Figure 10.9)

Repeat these actions three to five times, adding Lion Face Pose on the exhale.

To come out, exhale and release your arms to your sides.

Note: If you have difficulty taking your arms overhead, you can practice this exercise by raising your arms from your sides to shoulder height.

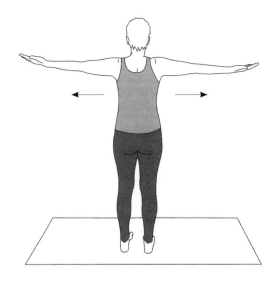

Figure 10.9: Broaden with both arms extended, palms up.

Core Action 2c: Connect

In this exercise we want the scapulae and the ribs to talk to one another a bit more, so they can work together in harmony. Your shoulder blades are continually gliding over your ribs without your realizing it. Your ribs provide a foundation for your scapulae, similar to how the floor provides a foundation for your feet. Applying this action brings a greater sense of connection between the ribs of your upper back and your shoulder blades. This connection is stabilizing to the shoulder joint.

As you explore the relationship between your shoulder blades and rib cage at your upper back, you may begin to notice that neither is a flat surface. Both have curves and nuances. Inviting the shoulder blades and ribs to support one another with awareness will bring stability, strength, and healthy flexibility to your upper back, shoulders, and chest, as well as lay a foundation for healthy head, neck, and jaw alignment.

The shoulder blades are naturally stabilized against the ribs when you push against an object. You can experience this by simply pushing against a wall.

EXERCISE: WALL PUSH

Props needed: A wall

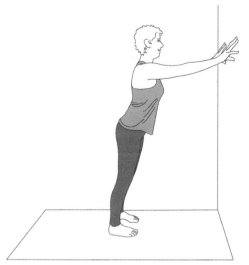

Face the wall and stand close enough to place your fingertips at shoulder height or just below, with your elbows bent. Step away from the wall to straighten your arms and lean lightly into the wall. Keep your body in one line. Now try to gently push the wall away. Keep your chest open and head lifted. Notice what your shoulder blades are doing. How do they feel against your back?

Note: Depending on your flexibility, there are a couple of approaches to connecting the shoulder blades to the upper back. Repeat the Wall Push exercise, experimenting with each of the following.

Figure 10.10: Straighten your arms, keeping your body in one line, and gently yet firmly push the wall with your fingertips.

■ APPROACH #1: PRESSING IN

If you are stiff, newer to yoga, or have a limited range of movement, focus on pressing the shoulder blades onto your back. This happens naturally when we push against an object as in the exercise above. Repeat the exercise to notice this action.

■ APPROACH #2: EXPANDING OUT

If you are more flexible, have practiced yoga for an extended period, or have hypermobile joints, a different approach can be helpful. Instead of pressing your shoulder blades onto your back, allow your back ribs to fill out—like plumping up a down feather pillow—and adhere them to your shoulder blades. Do this without rounding your upper back. This requires a bit more focus and clear intention. Try the previous exercise again with this possibility in mind.

EXERCISE: ARMS EXTENDED IN A T

Let's repeat the earlier Arms Extended in a T exercise with a new focus: connecting shoulders and ribs.

Stand with feet hip-width apart and arms at your sides. Inhale and raise your arms overhead as described in the Reach and Shrug exercise (page 126), then exhale and lower your shoulder blades and arms to shoulder height as in Both Arms Extended in a T (page 128). Now imagine pressing your shoulder blades onto your upper back as you expand your upper back to meet your shoulder blades. Maintain the lift of your upper sternum and openness of your chest. Add Lion Face Pose on the exhale. Hold for three breaths.

To come out, exhale and lower your arms to your sides.

Repeat the entire exercise three to five times, holding for three breaths each time.

Review and Refine: All Three Shoulder Actions

EXERCISE: PARTNER WORK

It is hard to touch or see your own upper back, so working with a partner can really help. Proprioception—the capacity to sense where your body is in space—can be developed through conscious touch and careful practice. Having a friend assist with the following exercise will deepen your awareness of the three shoulder blade actions. To review, these actions support opening of your upper chest, back, shoulders, and neck. When you practice this *with awareness of your jaw* through Lion Face Pose, you are reintegrating your jaw with the rest of your body and thus helping to unravel the habit of tension. As a result, these core actions lay a foundation for a more relaxed jaw.

Caution: It is important that your partner not try to move your shoulder blades for you or push so much that your posture is thrown off (i.e., you shouldn't feel pushed forward or pulled backward). Just the contact of their hands or the yoga block is enough.

Props needed: A friend

Optional props: One yoga block

Stand with your feet hip-width apart and arms at your sides. Have your friend stand behind you and place their hands or a yoga block on your shoulder blades (see figures 10.1 and 10.5 for locations of the shoulder blades).

Allow the feeling of the block or your friend's hands to inform you about the placement of your shoulder blades in your upper back as you practice each of the shoulder blade actions described above (*release*, *broaden*, and *connect*). Invite your friend to provide verbal feedback regarding the movement of your shoulder blades. For example, your friend may notice that one shoulder blade lifts and releases more easily, while the other side broadens more fully. See if their observations correspond with your inner experience: What do you notice?

Exercise: Shoulder Harness

In this exercise a yoga strap creates a support for accessing the three shoulder blade actions. The placement of the strap is important. Similar to working with a partner, the contact of the yoga belt on your body will help you to develop greater body awareness and proprioception. Take your time with getting into and out of this posture. Be sure there are no twists in the belt as this could pinch your skin and cause discomfort. The harness should feel supportive and comfortable. You might have your friend help you create the harness the first few times. With practice it becomes easier to do this on your own.

Props needed: Ten-foot yoga strap
Optional props: A friend

While standing, place the middle of the strap across your mid-upper back just below your shoulder blades. Keep this portion of the strap flat against your back. Wrap the strap under your armpits, around to the front of your body, and over your shoulders. Let the ends of the straps hang down your back. They should be fairly even in length. Reach back and tuck the loose ends under the portion of the strap that rests against your back. Cross the ends so they make an X just above where the strap rests against your back. Make sure there are no twists anywhere in the strap. (Figure 10.11)

Stand with your feet hip-width apart. Hold one end of the strap in each hand. Pull downward with equal pressure on each end. Allow the strap at the back of your body to tighten gently. With a steady pull on the ends, feel how the strap is teaching your shoulder blades to drop, broaden, and stabilize against your back, as well as encouraging you to lift your upper sternum. Do not arch your back. Allow the ribs of your upper back to expand. Observe the connection between your shoulder blades and the ribs of your upper back. Add Lion Face Pose on the exhale.

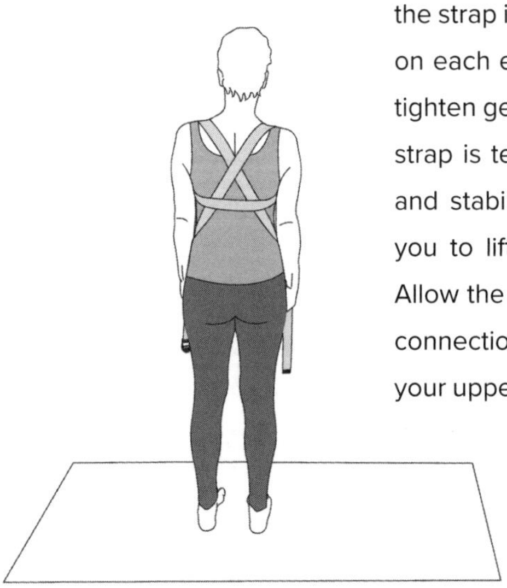

Figure 10.11: Shoulder harness.

Taking It Deeper: Revisiting the Body Map

Practicing the three actions of releasing, broadening, and stabilizing your shoulder blades most likely led you to new observations and insights. So let's update your personal body map.

As you explored your shoulders, did you notice which side is tighter? Which can access the actions more easily? Which has greater range of motion? Mark this information down on your body map.

Now look at the patterns that show up on your map. Is your tight shoulder on the same side that your jaw tends to be tight? And is this the side where you experience jaw pain, headaches, migraines? Is this also the side where you experience sacroiliac pain, hip pain, or sciatica? Or is it the opposite side? Take note of the patterns that you see and feel so you can track the changes that will happen as your practice continues.

Core Action 3: Hips

As we saw in part one, the pelvis and jaw are closely connected through the core link (figure 5.3). Thanks to this connection, we can relieve jaw tension through work with the hips. A key core action for our yoga practice is the rotation of the upper thighs. This action lays a foundation for almost all of the yoga poses in this program, especially the standing poses and hip openers. So let's explore the way the pelvis interrelates with the thighbones and spine, including sacrum and tailbone—focusing in particular on the rotation of the thighbones in the hip sockets.

The rotation of the femur (thighbone) is subtle but important. What we are looking for is not a big movement but rather a clear sense of how the top of the thigh rests and moves within the pelvis. Keep in mind that the head of your femur is about the size of your fist. Its placement can have a significant impact on the openness of the pelvis, the overall connection between the upper and lower body, and ultimately the jaw.

Ramanand Patel's careful investigation into the impact of internal versus external rotation of the upper thighs inspired me to cultivate awareness of this action in my daily life and activities. It is one of several aspects of yoga he taught that connected the dots between yoga and craniosacral. The movements resulting from femur rotation correspond to the inner tide as defined by Dr. William Sutherland, the founder of cranial osteopathy. We explored this subject in chapter 3. Femur rotation is one of the many subtle coordinated movements throughout the body corresponding to the health and well-being and maintenance of the human nervous system.

When we move the hips, we often externally rotate our thighs. Internal rotation is less common in day-to-day movements; for most people it requires specific intention. Dancers (particularly in ballet) will recognize this movement as part of their routine. It involves isolating the thigh rotation as distinct from the movement of the leg and foot—meaning your feet stay parallel even as your thighs rotate. Internal rotation will awaken the pelvic floor, relax the gluteus, and free the sacrum and tailbone. If you keep working with internal thigh rotation, it can free up your lower back and help reclaim the natural curves of your spine—and even balance your shoulders, arms, and head in their positions relative to the rest of your body. Eventually this core action can become a gentle whole-body dance that reintegrates body and mind. Let's proceed step by step.

There should be no strain in your joints when you practice these actions. Your hips, knees, and ankles should feel at ease. Your knee and ankle joints will move slightly with the rotation of your thighbones, but it should not cause discomfort. If you have tight joints, this action may initially be difficult to access. If you have loose joints, do less. Do not cause strain, instability, or over-stretching. The pelvis will follow along, in response to rotation of the thighbones.

EXERCISE: BLOCK SQUEEZE AND RELEASE

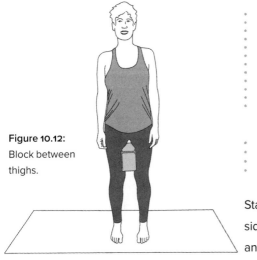

Figure 10.12:
Block between
thighs.

Caution: If you experience discomfort in your joints, stop what you are doing. Stand or walk for a minute, then try again. See if you can use a little less effort and still allow the thighbones to rotate. Remember to breathe.

Props needed: Thick foam block (4 x 6 x 9 inches)

Stand with your feet hip-width apart and the outsides of your feet parallel. Lift your toes, lengthen and spread them, then place your toes back on the floor, retaining the length and spread. Place the short skinny side of your block comfortably between your thighs, positioned so it sticks out above your knees. Firm your thighs, without squeezing the block. (See Standing Mountain Pose on page 147 for more detailed information on how to stand.)

Note: For many people there is a temptation to squeeze the block, so take a few seconds to intentionally squeeze it, and then consciously relax. Try to relax enough so that the thighs are toned but not gripping. Imagine releasing your thighbones away from the block. This will allow your pelvic floor muscles to relax.

If the muscles running down your inner thighs (adductors) are hard, or if you feel tightness in the inner groin (psoas insertion), a lot of pressure on the block, or a headache, *these are all signs you are squeezing the block more than necessary.* Too much squeezing can interfere with the rotation of your thighs. If you find it difficult to stop squeezing the block, simply focus on squeezing and relaxing for a while. Then walk around for a minute, and try again. Be patient. The results will be worth it. It's important the pelvic floor muscles stay relaxed in this exercise.

EXERCISE: THIGH ROTATION WITH BLOCK

Props needed: Thick foam block (4 x 6 x 9 inches)

Purposefully place the block a little forward between your thighs. Bend your knees a little. Roll your thighbones toward each other (internal rotation) and notice the block move backward. Roll your thighbones away from each other

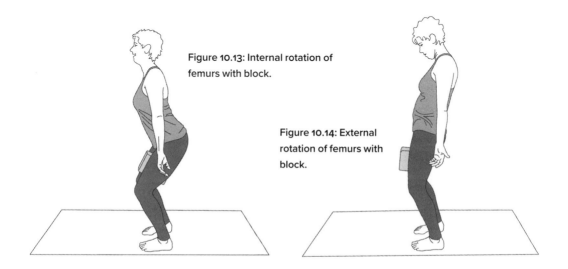

Figure 10.13: Internal rotation of femurs with block.

Figure 10.14: External rotation of femurs with block.

(external rotation); notice the block move forward. Allow your pelvis to move in response to the rotation of your thighs.

Watching the movement of the block is one way to gain confidence in your thigh rotation. Another way is to feel the contact of your muscles against the block. As your thighs roll toward one another (internal rotation), you feel more of the front inner thigh contacting the block. As your thighs roll away from one another (external rotation), you feel the back inner thigh contacting the block more. Practice this for two to three minutes, rotating the thighs slowly, paying close attention to the sensation of your thighs contacting the block. Add Lion Face Pose on an exhale.

Note: If you are having difficulty, you may be using either too much or too little effort. Let's look at how to find just the right amount.

Too much tension in your belly or buttocks makes it difficult to access these gentle movements. With your hand, gently poke your butt and notice: Does it feel hard? If so, you are working too hard. Try to let your gluteus muscles relax. Now let's do the same with your belly. Does it feel hard to the touch? See if you can soften your belly. Three-Part Breathing (page 212) can help.

The gluteus muscles should fire up as you move through internal and external rotation, but keeping your butt clenched will get in the way. Similarly, the lower abdominal muscles (rectus abdominis) will activate as a part of this action, but holding your belly in and overworking the abdominals will interfere with your capacity to rotate your thighbones. Overworking or underworking in the pelvic floor also make thigh rotation difficult.

EXERCISE: THIGH ROTATION WITHOUT THE BLOCK

Once you are able to access the rotation of your femurs, try it without the block between the thighs. For some this exercise may be easier than the version with the block.

Caution: There should be no pain in your knee and ankle joints. If pain arises in these joints, stop. Stand and breathe. Try again with a smaller movement, letting the movement originate from your upper thigh bones.

Stand with feet hip-width apart and the outsides of your feet parallel. Lift your toes, lengthen and spread them, and place them back on the floor maintaining the length and spread. Bend your knees just a little. Become aware of the heads of your thighbones resting in your hips. Gently begin to rotate your thighbones toward one another (internal rotation), noticing how your legs respond to this action. Then gently rotate your thighbones away from one another (external rotation), once again noticing how your legs respond.

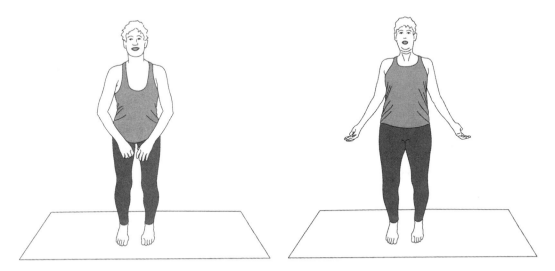

Figure 10.15: Internal femur rotation without block.   Figure 10.16: External femur rotation without block.

Now match the rotations to your breathing. On the exhale, rotate your thighbones inward. On the inhale, rotate them outward. Continue until it feels natural, so there is less effort to coordinate the breath and thighbone rotation. Allow the breath to just flow. Slow down and enjoy the experience of your body moving through its natural cycles of expansion and release.

Now observe how your pelvis responds to the gentle internal and external rotation of your thighbones. Allow your pelvis to move. Trying to force your pelvis to stay still will interfere with this action. Notice how your spine and torso respond to the rotation of your femurs. Notice your arms and shoulders. Notice the gentle movement in your neck and head in response to the rotation of your femurs.

A gentle rotation of your thighbones can get your whole body moving with a wavelike motion. This wavelike movement will naturally become coordinated with the breath when you are in a relaxed state. It may begin to feel like a dance, at times growing larger or smaller. Allow yourself to enjoy this movement. Investigate this motion for two or three minutes.

▦ PELVIS AND SACRUM AWARENESS

As you continue rotating your thighbones in and out, let your pelvis move in response. Do not try to keep the pelvis fixed. Likewise allow your spine and torso to move. Reconnect to the femur rotation as the origin of any movement in your body at this time, and notice the ripples that spread through your body as you stand and practice this gentle movement.

Imagine you can lift your pelvis up off your thighbones. Notice what happens. Do you take a deeper breath?

Investigate what happens to your sacrum, tailbone, and pelvis as you internally and externally rotate your thighs. As the thighbones *externally* rotate, the pelvis tucks under. The weight moves to the outer feet. The pubis lifts, and the sacrum drops. The sacrum is compressed as the pelvic bones move toward each other at the back of the body and away from each other at the front of the body (the belly). When thighbones *internally* rotate, the pelvis untucks. The weight falls more to the inner feet—the arches, big toe, and inner heel. The sacrum and pelvic bones lift at the back of the body and drop at the front of the body. There is more space around the sacrum as the pelvic bones move away from the sacrum at the back of the body and toward each other across the abdomen.

▦ SPINE, TORSO, AND HEAD AWARENESS

What happens to the curves of your spine as the thighbones rotate and the pelvis tucks and untucks? For example, can you detect a ripple effect up through your torso, neck, and head? See if you can perceive the spinal curves increasing and decreasing (flattening), the subtle lift of the chest with the simultaneous drop of the upper back—and the reverse, an expansion of the upper back accompanied by a dropping or contracting of the chest. Does the ripple of movement include your neck and head? You may begin to perceive your body differently, noticing what feels free and what feels tight or restricted.

As you practice the thigh rotation exercises, you may begin to sense differences between the right and left sides of your body. This is a good sign. Don't try to correct these right away. Just consider these observations to be information about what happens in your body. It's very likely that one leg will be able to rotate more. Notice which side it is. Grow curious about the differences. No one has a perfectly balanced body. We all have subtle or gross right-left patterns of restriction and movement. Rushing to correct them can cause more difficulty. Over time, as we learn to work more skillfully with our body patterns, we will experience true release and greater freedom of movement.

Taking It Deeper: Revisiting the Body Map

As you play with the thigh rotation and full body wave, take a few minutes to update your body map with the new insights you gain into your right-left tension patterns and range of motion in your joints.

Core Action 4: Feet

Within your body, nothing could be farther from your jaw than your feet. And yet they are a part of the same body and *are* interconnected. Your feet create the foundation for your standing posture, impacting your legs, hips, and torso and even your head, neck, and jaw. This subject is explored more fully in part one of this book, including how bunions can be caused by neck and jaw tension (chapter 7).

I have personal experience with how powerful precise foot work can be. When I first began to walk, my parents noticed I was pigeon-toed. My right foot, in particular, turned in. I was born in the era of metal leg braces for correcting pronation, but luckily my pediatrician was a bit of a hippie. She recommended to my parents that whenever possible I not wear shoes as an infant, thinking that the extra weight of the shoes might contribute to increasing the pronation. As a result, I was a barefoot baby and toddler. I never got a pair of the leather oxford baby shoes that were so common in the late 1960s. I did however have a slight pronation throughout my adolescence, which probably contributed to knee pain when I began to run a lot in high school (including both indoor and outdoor track for a couple of years).

In 1996 I moved to San Francisco and began to practice yoga with Ramanand Patel. Through him I learned a very careful and detailed approach to working with the feet. His approach helped me understand the connection between the feet, legs, and hips. After one year of working in this way, I was no longer pigeon-toed. This tendency only returns occasionally, when I feel like a neglected child. At those times I am feeling vulnerable, and I recognize it as a sign to hold myself with tenderness and compassion.

As you begin practicing the core actions devoted to your feet, don't worry if they are difficult. Try to have a sense of play in this investigation. We are learning about cause and effect in the body—how one movement or action has an effect on another part of the body or mind. You are gaining information about your feet, how you stand, and the differences between right and left sides. This is a way of training your mind and body to perceive subtlety.

Your feet are your earth connection. They keep you grounded and connected. Bringing more attention to your feet can help you to feel more at ease anywhere. Imagine your feet are like the roots of a tree. The roots, sunk into the earth, anchor the tree even in heavy storms. The tree is very much a part of the community and the environment in which it resides. The roots allow the tree to grow up, stand tall, spread its branches, grow leaves, and bear fruit. You can apply the practices introduced here throughout your day. Every time you stand up, take a moment to notice your feet.

This work will be further developed in chapter 11, particularly in Standing Mountain Pose (page 147) and other standing poses.

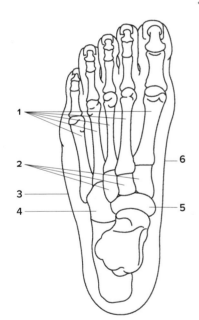

Figure 10.17: Anatomy of the foot.

1. metatarsals   **4.** cuboid
2. cuneiforms   **5.** navicular
3. outer arch   **6.** inner arch

EXERCISE: WORKING WITH YOUR ROOTS

Stand with your feet hip-width apart and your toes spread as widely open as possible. Take a deep breath and exhale with a sigh. Allow your face to soften. Allow your body to release unnecessary tension. Notice that the outer feet are pressing down, while the inner feet are both *pressing down* (at toes and heels) *and lifting up* (at arches).

OUTER FOOT AWARENESS

Bring attention to your outer foot contacting the floor. Imagine a line from your pinkie toe to your heel, and notice whether there are gaps—places along that line where your outer foot and the floor do not touch. Experiment with trying to make this line continuous, so there is a steady contact from pinkie toe to heel.

INNER FOOT AWARENESS

Bring your attention to your inner foot. Imagine a line from your big toe to your heel. Track the length of this line, noticing where your feet are contacting the floor and where there is no contact due to the arches. Notice the difference between your right and left foot. Is one arch higher or longer? Experiment to see whether you can lift your arch without displacing your ankle right or left. Keep your ankle directly above your heel and your heel in line with your knee.

FINDING YOUR ARCHES

To work more precisely with the arches and soles of the feet, let's divide them up into quadrants for your awareness. With your mind's eye, draw three lines across the sole of your foot, from inner foot to outer foot: the first is drawn where the arch begins, a little below the ball of the foot; the next is at the highest point of the arch; the third is just in front of the heel, where the arch ends. These lines give a focus for your attention. Let your mind follow these lines while notic- ing the quality of feeling in your arches.

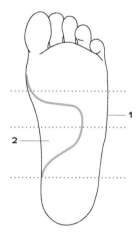

Figure 10.18: Sole of foot with arch. The dotted lines define the top, middle, and bottom of the arch.

1. outer arch
2. inner arch

How does each of these areas of your foot feel? Does the arch feel vaulted, or collapsed? Is it overly activated or rigid? Notice dif- ferences between your right and left feet. This might feel weird at first. Take your time and be patient. With practice, it will become eas- ier. Eventually you can feel the continuity of the arch on each foot, where it is properly vaulted, and where it is either tight or loose. Gently working to create a balance in your feet through this practice will bring changes in how you stand, the feeling of being grounded and connected, and in your overall body structure.

WHOLE BODY AWARENESS: STANDING MEDITATION

Notice sensations throughout your body and changes in your mind as you stand with awareness of your feet. Sense the earth beneath the floor, in essence supporting you. Become aware of your connection to—and dependence on— Mother Earth.

Feel the weight of your body dropping through your feet into the earth. Sense that even as you push down, Mother Earth pushes back up through your feet. Whether you are aware of it or not, she is there providing support and nourish- ment. This is a dynamic relationship, full of vitality and nutriment. This connection is available to you at any moment throughout all of your days and nights here on planet earth. It can be grounding and calming to return to this during the busy-ness of your day, even for a minute or two.

Notice what changes in your mind as you envision your connection with the earth. Perhaps thoughts fall away, small sounds suddenly seem louder, or the noise of life disappears and you are enveloped by a deep quiet. You may become aware of different aches, pains, or restrictions throughout your body. This is a good sign. It means body, mind, and heart are starting to come into bal-ance in a new way. Understanding this may help you to respond rather than react to what you are experiencing.

As we continue to explore, remember that you can always come back to these basic principles—breathing with ease, letting go of unnecessary tension, stand-ing with more lightness, and feeling your connection to the earth.

$\textcolor{gray}{\diamondsuit}$11

Yoga Poses

I N THIS CHAPTER we will integrate the four core actions from chapter 10 into yoga poses. Performing yoga poses regularly can help build greater awareness of body tension patterns and reduce jaw tension and its resulting repercussions. When practicing yoga, it's very important to listen inwardly to your body. If you are new to yoga, you will likely experience new sensations that may be uncomfortable at first. Remember to breathe. Soften. Explore. Grow curious. Are the sensations you're feeling harmful or beneficial? It isn't always easy to tell immediately; this is where working with a qualified yoga teacher can be pragmatic. Learning to mindfully observe and consider your reactions can be profoundly transformative. Engage the principle of ehi-passiko and get closer to trusting your own deepest knowing as you explore the beautiful practice of yoga.

1. CAT/DOG POSE

This gentle pose is a great way to begin to move your spine and feel the connection between your head and tail, known as the *core link* (figure 5.3) in craniosacral. It can also provide an introduction to the inner tide (chapter 3) when done slowly, coordinated with your breathing. Once you are familiar with this pose, be like a fly on the wall, observing what happens in your body as you practice it. Can you feel the way your femurs (thighbones) and humeri (upper arm bones) rotate in response to the movements of your spine and pelvis? This is more of an action than a movement, which means it's subtle and happens naturally, without your trying.

Caution: If you have slipped or ruptured discs, or spondylolisthesis, do not arch your back. Go between neutral spine and rounding.

Props needed: Yoga mat

Optional props: Folded blanket (for cushioning under your knees)

Begin on your hands and knees: hands below your shoulders, knees under your hips and hip-width apart. Spread your fingers wide and extend them fully. Press down at the base of the fingers, particularly the index fingers. Notice your breathing. Imagine you have a tail. Move from tail to head, coordinating this movement with your breathing. Breathing in, lift your tail, drop your navel, open your chest, and lift your head, allowing your back to arch. Breathing out, drop your tail, lift your navel, round your back, and drop your head. Take your time. Explore each portion of the movement. As you continue, allow your breath to lead the movement. Repeat for one minute.

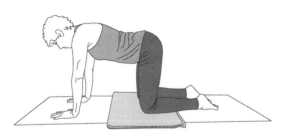

Figure 11.1: Cat/Dog Pose with neutral spine.

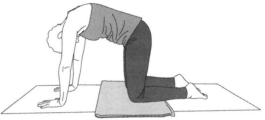

Figure 11.2: Cat/Dog Pose with tail lifted.

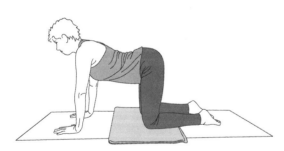

Figure 11.3: Cat/Dog Pose with tail dropped.

Notes: This pose is great for experiencing the inner tide as well as core actions of the hips and shoulders. Rather than trying to engage the actions, instead notice how the oscillation of your spine invites the rotation of your limbs. Allow the scapulae to glide up and down in response to the spinal movement. The shoulder actions of releasing, broadening, and connecting occur on the inhale. Relax your jaw. Do not strain your neck. Lift your head only as much as feels comfortable. If your knees are sore, try pressing your shins down onto the floor to more evenly distribute your weight. If your wrists are sore, you can make a gentle fist with your hands, placing your knuckles on the ground for support. This keeps your wrists neutral.

2. Puppy Pose

Named for a puppy ready to play, this pose is a great way to begin to open up your back body—hips, shoulders, and the length of your arms.

Props needed: Yoga mat
Optional props: Folded blanket (for cushioning under your knees)

Begin on hands and knees as in Cat/ Dog Pose (figure 11.1), this time with your feet near the end of your mat. Curl your toes under. Exhaling, push your buttocks back toward your feet. Then stretch your hands and arms forward as far as you can *without lifting your hips*. Keep your arms

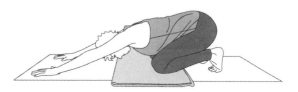

Figure 11.4: Puppy Pose.

straight and long. Press your hands and fingers down onto your mat. Keep your arms and shoulders active and lifted off of your mat. Keep your head neutral, in line with your arms. This is Puppy Pose. Breathe slowly. Stay here for three to five breaths. Enjoy the stretch as you feel your body start to open up.

3. Child's Pose (Balasana)

Child's Pose is a resting pose. It is calming and soothing as it puts your spine in flexion and offers a bit of sense withdrawal. If you do not have the flexibility to practice this pose with ease initially, try placing a yoga block under your head or a bolster under your torso. It's important your belly and torso are able to rest in this pose. Make sure the tops of your feet are on the ground (as opposed to toes curled under).

Props needed: Yoga mat
Optional props: Folded blanket (to cushion your knees), yoga block (for your head), bolster (to support torso)

Begin on hands and knees as in Cat/Dog Pose (figure 11.1). Exhaling, bring your feet together, and lower your buttocks to your heels, your belly to your thighs and forehead to the floor. Your arms may rest on the floor overhead or extended

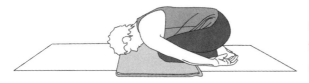

at your sides with palms up. Stay here for one minute or more—as long as is comfortable.

Figure 11.5: Child's Pose. You can also extend your arms on the floor above your head if you prefer.

Note: If your forehead does not easily reach the floor, rest it on a block. If your hips do not easily reach your heels or your belly doesn't rest on your thighs, place a bolster lengthwise under your torso for support. If you are not comfortable, then it will be difficult to relax. Take a few minutes to modify the pose to meet your needs.

4. DOWNWARD DOG POSE (ADHO MUKHA SVANASANA)

Downward Dog Pose is beneficial in our work with jaw tension for several reasons. Shoulder and neck tension are common repercussions of chronic clenching or grinding. There are direct connections between the neck, jaw, and pelvis (figure 7.1). This pose opens the shoulders, lengthens the spine, extends the legs, and begins to open the hips. In addition Downward Dog is a gateway to many of the arm-supported inverted poses. It helps build strength, stability, and healthy alignment in the upper body if practiced with wise attention.

Props needed: Yoga mat
Optional props: Folded blanket (to cushion your knees), block (for your head)

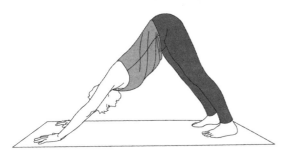

Begin from Puppy Pose (figure 11.4). Keep your hands and feet where they are as you exhale, lift your hips, straighten your arms, release your hips back, and lift up onto your toes with knees bent. Keep your head in line with your arms. Now begin to straighten your legs by pressing your heels down. Stay for three to five breaths initially. Stay longer as you feel more comfortable in the pose.

Figure 11.6: Downward Dog Pose.

To come out: Go to Child's Pose (figure 11.5): Exhaling, bend both knees and bring them back to the floor, resting on hands and knees. Take a breath in. On your next exhale, bring your feet together, then lower your hips to your heels and forehead to the floor. Your arms rest on the floor overhead or at your sides with palms up. If your forehead does not easily reach the floor, rest your forehead on a block.

Note: While in Downward Dog, apply the core action for shoulders (page 124, figure 10.3): release, broaden, and connect. Apply the core action for hips (page 122, figure 10.1): femur rotation with awareness. Notice how the femurs are resting in the pelvis. Is your tail released? In most cases gentle internal rotation helps to release the tail, external rotation can cause compression. Experiment with bending and straightening alternate legs, one at a time, to pay closer attention to the femur. Feel how it changes as you straighten your leg(s). Apply the jaw core action (page 124, figure 10.2) of Lion Face Pose.

5. STANDING MOUNTAIN POSE (TADASANA)

Standing Mountain Pose lays the foundation for all other poses, whether they are standing, seated, supine, or inverted. It is a formal yoga pose, but it can also inform us on how to be present in the world. You might try practicing Mountain Pose throughout your day—when you are standing in line, washing dishes, or while on the train or bus. Standing, breathing, aware—both alert and calm, deeply within our own being, and yet receptive. Standing poses all begin in Mountain Pose. *All of the core actions will be incorporated in this pose.*

The anatomical explanations in part one and the core actions in chapter 10 helped to clarify how your jaw is connected with the rest of your body. Standing Mountain Pose gives you an opportunity to work skillfully with these cross-connections. Begin by observing your experience as you follow the instructions.

Resist the temptation to "fix things" right away. As your yoga practice deepens, the pathway to positive change will become clear. And here's a little secret: By simply noticing cause and effect, something has already begun to change. You are on the healing path. Remember to play with the information presented below. Don't worry about getting it "right" but rather enjoy the exploration.

Standing, place your feet hip-width apart, with the outsides of your feet parallel. Feel how the weight of your body drops through your feet into the floor. Imagine a line running from the crown of your head down through your feet. Find a

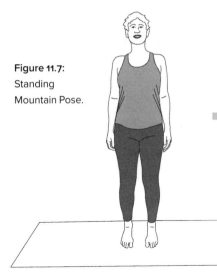

posture of stability, like a mountain. Continue to develop the pose by applying the core actions, as detailed below. Stay for one minute or longer.

■ FOOT AWARENESS—CORE ACTION 4 (PAGE 139)

Widen the balls of the feet. To do this, lift your toes. Bring the big toes back to the floor while keeping your other toes lifted. Widen the base of your big toes. You should feel an increase of contact with the floor in this area. Widen the base of your other toes by spreading your lifted toes as wide as possible before placing them back on the floor, maintaining the spread. Do not grip the floor or hold unnecessary tension in your toes.

If your toes don't spread out on their own, you can bend over and use your fingers to spread them. Don't worry if they don't want to spread out or if they close up again once you take your hands away. Over time your feet will be more able to hold the adjustment, and spreading your toes will become easier.

■ LEG AND HIP AWARENESS—CORE ACTION 3 (PAGE 133)

Bend your knees slightly. Lift your pelvis as if it could float above your thighs. Allow your spine to find its natural curves. When the pelvis is tucked under, the curve in the lower back is lost, causing strain in the muscles. When the pelvis is pushed back, there can be too much curve in the lower back, causing instability and weakness. The thigh rotations of this core action will help you to find the correct placement of your hips and the right amount of spinal curve.

■ RIB, SHOULDER, AND JAW AWARENESS—CORE ACTIONS 2 (PAGE 124) AND 1 (PAGE 122)

Lift your rib cage as though it could float above your pelvis. Feel the gentle expansion and release of your ribs as you breathe in and out. Allow your shoulders to balance above your ribs and let your arms rest at your sides. *Remember the three-part shoulder core action:* Lift the top of your sternum; then release, broaden, and connect your shoulder blades. Notice this gives a lift to your neck and head. Think of a plumb line from the crown of your head hanging down through the center of your body and allow your feet, hips, shoulders, and head to come into a vertical line. Applying Lion Face Pose (page 124) reminds you to relax your jaw and supports finding this vertical plumb line.

▪ Eye Awareness

Keep your eyes level with the horizon. If your eyes are dropped or lifted, this will impact your head and in turn cause strain in your neck and jaw. Soften your gaze. Let your eyes rest back into your head.

Note: As you find the inner vertical line in Mountain Pose, you may notice that your mind becomes quiet. There is less chatter. Perhaps you naturally take a deeper breath. These are good signs. You may want to experiment with a small "dance"—swaying a tiny bit forward and backward and then side to side to find your vertical line. Allow the swaying to settle into stillness and stability.

6. Wide Leg Pose (Padottanasana)

Wide Leg Pose is the foundation of all of the standing poses that follow, and it helps our work with jaw tension in a variety of ways. This pose builds strength and stability in the legs, opens the hips, is grounding, and is accessible to many. It is a balanced pose, so we can more easily perceive differences in the right and left sides of the body—especially the hips.

We will practice Wide Leg Pose in two stages. The first has slightly bent knees to facilitate the rotation of our thighbones. In the second stage, we straighten our legs without locking or hyper-extending the knees.

Caution: Rotating your thighbones should not hurt your knees or ankles. If your knee or ankle joints become sore, try rotating in a smaller range and focus on the femur head. Do less. If needed, come out of the pose by stepping your feet together. Stand and breathe. Walk around the room for a minute. Then try again.

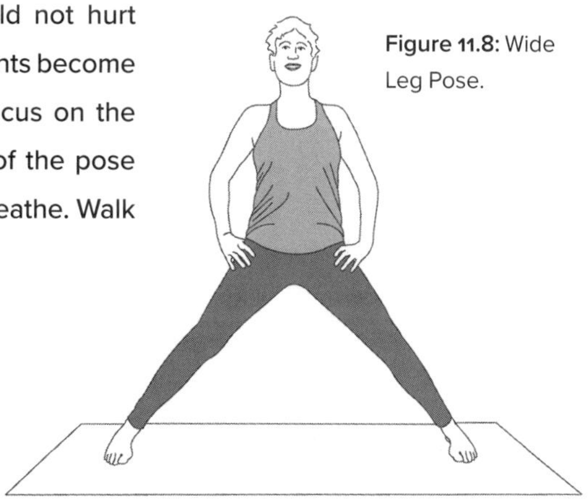

Figure 11.8: Wide Leg Pose.

Props needed: Yoga mat (optional)

Stand in Mountain Pose (figure 11.7). Exhaling, step your feet four to four and a half feet apart, keeping the outsides of your outer feet parallel.

Place your hands on your outer hips at your groin crease, where your thighs join your pelvis. Stay here for three to five breaths initially.

FEET—CORE ACTION 4 (PAGE 139)

Bend your knees just a little. Notice how your weight falls through your feet and how your feet contact the floor. Press down a bit more on your outer feet, bringing the outer line of your foot toward the floor while lifting on your inner feet, aware of the inner line of your foot. Notice the lift of your arches and contact at toes and heels. Remember the three lines of awareness across the arches of your feet. Notice which of these arches are relatively easy to access and where your foot has difficulty working. Is it the same on the right and left sides or different? Draw a map in your mind of which areas are harder to access on each foot.

FEMUR ROTATION WITH BENT KNEES—CORE ACTION 3 (PAGE 133)

With your knees slightly bent, begin to rotate your femurs in and out gently. This movement should originate at the upper portion or head of the thighbone, where it rests into the pelvis. Remember, the actual movement is small. We are focused on the intention to create a specific action rather than trying to generate a lot of movement.

Notice the effect this action has on your hips, sacrum, and breath. Are you holding your breath? Remember to breathe freely.

INTEGRATING HIPS, TORSO, AND SPINE

Once you are comfortable with femur rotation, let your body awareness expand to notice how this action influences the length of your spine, including back, shoulders, neck, head, and jaw. It may be helpful to close your eyes to experience the sensations internally. When our eyes are open, they are usually focused on an object, which can interfere with and influence head movement. Closed eyes may allow your head to move more freely. You can also try softening your eyes and turning your gaze inward. Be less interested in seeing what is around you and more on your inner experience.

■ JAW—CORE ACTION 1 (PAGE 122)

Open your mouth and exhale, repeating Lion Face Pose three to five times. Notice the effect on your jaw.

■ STAGE 2: STRAIGHT LEGS

Allow the subtle movements you have been working with to settle down, and let your body come to stillness while standing in Wide Leg Pose. Keep your hands at your groin crease, where your thighs join your pelvis. Straighten your legs by lifting your knees and thighs while pressing down through your feet. What happens to the heads of your thighbones in your pelvis? Notice if they jump forward, or there is a feeling of hardening in the inner groin or pelvis. Bend your knees just a little and then straighten. Repeat three to five times, paying close attention to what happens in your hip sockets as your legs straighten.

■ FEMUR HEADS

See if you can keep a spacious quality in your pelvis, length in your inner groin, openness in the hip sockets. Does a very gentle rotation of your femur facilitate this? In most cases a slight internal rotation will help to stabilize and open the pelvis. But this is not always true, since everyone has a slightly different pelvis. Notice what works for you. Perhaps internal rotation on one side and external rotation on the other? Or is it something else?

Observe which side of your pelvis you feel you access easily and which one is more challenging for you. Is there one hip that moves more easily? Keep this in mind as we'll come back to it when we activate our shoulders.

■ PELVIS, SPINE, AND TORSO

Lift your pelvis, as though it could float up off your thighbones. Releasing the psoas muscle attachments at the lesser trochanter on your inner upper thigh will support this. Feel that your back is long and your pelvis is balanced over your legs and feet, not tilting overly forward or backward. Lengthen your spine. Lift your ribs, as though they can float up away from your pelvis. Open your chest and upper back. Lift your sternum and lengthen up through the top of your head.

▪ SHOULDERS: ARMS OVERHEAD—CORE ACTION 2 (PAGE 124)

To bring your arms into this pose, first reach your arms overhead (figure 10.6 without strap), then out to the sides. Refer to the variation of Arms Extended in a T (figure 10.9) if you need to refresh your memory.

Experiment with bending your knees slightly as you release your arms down on the exhale and straightening your legs as your raise your arms overhead on the inhale. Notice which of the shoulder actions—release, broaden, connect—you feel you access easily and which are more challenging for you. Does one shoulder move more easily? Is your stiff shoulder on the same side of your body or the opposite of your stiff hip? As you practice this regularly over time, notice whether the side that tends to be stiff changes. Allow yourself to be curious and enjoy the process rather than simply looking for results.

To come out: Exhaling, release your arms to your sides. Inhaling, step your feet together. Stand in Mountain Pose.

7. WARRIOR 2 POSE (VIRABHADRASANA 2)

Warrior 2 Pose is excellent for learning more about the uniqueness of your body. As we've seen, no one has a perfectly balanced body. We all have differences between our right and left sides, especially in the hips. This may not be readily apparent to everyone, but it's something we start to notice when we pay attention. The same is true for our mouth and jaw: as the Mirror Exercise (page 207) shows, the right and left sides are bound to be different.

Warrior 2 Pose is especially useful in our work with jaw tension because the right and left hips are doing different things (i.e., this pose opens the hips one at a time). There is a direct connection between your jaw and your hips. Opening the hips can help release your jaw, if appropriate awareness is applied. As you practice this pose, observe which hip is more open, which is tighter, which is more painful, and which is stabler. Which side of your jaw tends to be tighter? Is it the same side as your tight hip or the opposite side? Keep paying attention.

Using a wall is helpful in this pose. Placing your outer foot against a wall supports proprioception (knowing where you are in space) and gives information regarding how to work more effectively with feet and legs.

Caution: For the purpose of working with jaw tension, do not turn your head in this pose. Keeping your head neutral will facilitate experiencing the link between the jaw and upper neck as described in Guzay's theorem.

Props needed: Yoga mat, a wall

Place the yoga mat with its short end at the wall. Stand in the center of your mat in Mountain Pose. Step your feet four to four and a half feet apart to Wide Leg Pose (figure 11.8). Have the outside of your left foot at the wall. Rotate your left femur slightly in, in order to turn your left toes about thirty degrees away from the wall. Turn your right leg out ninety degrees, rotating from the top of your right thigh. Exhaling, bend the right knee ninety degrees so the shin and thigh form a right angle. Stay here for three to five breaths initially.

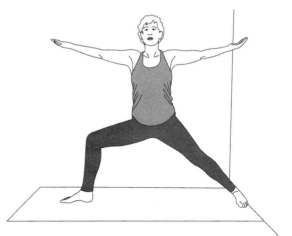

Figure 11.9: Warrior 2 Pose with a heel to the wall. Keep your head and neck neutral. Do not turn your head.

■ ARMS AND SHOULDERS—CORE ACTION 2 (PAGE 124)

Inhale and reach your arms overhead with palms facing each other, drawing your shoulders up close to your ears. To bring your arms down, let your shoulders lead the movement. Exhaling, release your shoulder blades down and away from each other. As your arms and shoulders move down, simultaneously lift your sternum. Keep your arms straight and stretch through your fingertips, broadening your upper back and chest. Lower your arms to shoulder height. Now allow your shoulder blades to connect to the ribs at the back of your body. Stay here for three to five breaths.

■ JAW—CORE ACTION 1 (PAGE 122)

Maintaining Warrior 2 Pose, add Lion Face Pose: exhaling, open your mouth, extend your tongue, relax your jaw, and free your TMJs.

To come out: Inhaling, straighten your legs and turn your feet to face forward. Exhaling, step your feet together and release your arms. Stand in Mountain Pose. Breathe. Repeat on the other side.

Troubleshooting: Does your sacrum feel compressed once you are in the full pose? Here's a way to free up your lower back as you enter Warrior 2. Starting with your right leg extending into the room and left foot at the wall, stand in Wide Leg Pose with legs straight and feet facing forward (figure 11.8). Place your left hand on your right outer hip bone (iliac crest). As you turn your foot and externally rotate your right leg, sweep your hand from your hip across your belly toward your navel. Through touch, you are giving your hip bone a sense of direction and inviting a little space into the sacroiliac joint.

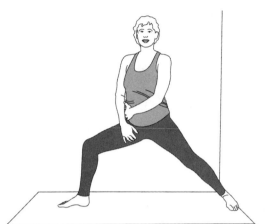

Now try it again, but this time also place your right hand at your groin crease—the place where your thigh joins your hip—with your thumb toward the inner groin and your other fingers toward your outer hip. As you externally rotate your leg, slide your hand toward your outer leg. This conscious touch gives your thigh a sense of direction, supporting external rotation. Repeat two to three times.

Figure 11.10: Warrior 2 Pose with the release of the sacroilliac joint. Use a gentle sweeping contact for release. Arrows indicate direction.

Take a moment to breathe in and out before going into the full pose. If these actions were helpful, they can be repeated as you bend your right knee to go into the full pose. Do not repeat if they were not helpful.

8. SIDE ANGLE POSE (PARSHVA KONASANA)

Side Angle Pose continues the journey of opening the hips one at a time and adds in side bending. In this pose your right and left arms and shoulders are doing different things at the same time, which is always good for your brain but can be challenging initially. Side Angle Pose is an excellent pose for releasing jaw tension as you deepen your practice. Practicing at the wall is helpful as it gives a contact for your outer foot and assists with orientation.

Props needed: Yoga mat, 2 yoga blocks

Place the yoga mat with its short end at the wall. Stand in Mountain Pose (figure 11.7). Step your feet four to four and a half feet apart with the outsides of your feet parallel in Wide Leg Pose (figure 11.8), placing the outside of your left foot at the wall. Rotate your left femur in slightly, turning your left toes in about thirty degrees. Rotate your right leg out ninety degrees. Exhaling, bend your right knee ninety degrees, so your shin and thigh form a right angle. Level your pelvis into Warrior 2 (figure 11.9). Notice whether there is any tension at the sacrum or sacroiliac joints. If there is, see the modification above (figure 11.10).

Inhaling, lengthen through your torso and the top of your head. Place your hands at your groin crease, where your thighs join your hips. Exhaling, extend your torso to your right, with the right side of your torso parallel to your right thigh. Stay here for three to five breaths initially.

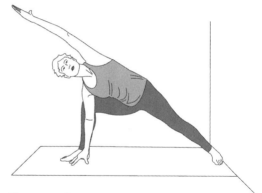

Figure 11.11: Side Angle Pose. Placing your back leg's heel at the wall brings stability.

◼ ARMS AND SHOULDERS—CORE ACTION 2 (PAGE 124)

Extend your right arm, placing your right hand on the floor, inside of your right thigh. (If it's difficult to reach the floor, use a yoga block.) Gently press your right upper arm against your right thigh. This serves as a reminder to keep your knee over your ankle on the bent-leg side. This can help protect the joints and open your hip. Release your right shoulder blade down, broadening your back and connecting with the ribs at the back of your body. Keep your chest open with your sternum lifted.

Swing your left arm in front of your body, elevating the shoulder blade and extending through your fingers. Bring your arm beside your head. Broaden your upper back and chest, and connect your shoulder blade and back ribs.

◼ HEAD

Keep your head in line with your sternum and lifted. Do not turn or drop your head; this can impact the neck or play into right-left imbalances in neck and jaw tension. Allow your neck to lengthen equally on both sides. Your right shoulder blade is released and your left is elevated.

On the side with the lowered arm (right side initially), try not to lean heavily on your hand or arm but rather slightly lift your torso away from that hand. On the side with the lifted arm (left arm initially), your shoulder and ear should feel spacious even as they align close to one another. Gently internally rotate your raised arm from the humerus (upper arm bone).

▪ JAW—CORE ACTION 1 (PAGE 122)

Add Lion Face Pose: exhaling, open your mouth, extend your tongue, relax your jaw, and free your TMJs.

To come out, inhale and reach your left arm up, returning to standing with your torso upright, arms extended out from your shoulders, and legs straight. Exhaling, turn your feet to face forward and release your arms. Step your feet together. Stand in Mountain Pose. Breathe. Repeat on the other side.

Troubleshooting: Does your sacrum feel compressed once you are in the full pose with your front knee bent? It may help to invite the iliac crest to release away from the sacrum, freeing it at the back body. To do this, repeat the Warrior 2 modification (figure 11.10) before moving into the final pose.

Begin in Wide Leg Pose with legs straight and feet facing forward. Place your left hand on your right outer hip bone (iliac crest). As you turn your right leg, sweep your left hand across your belly toward your navel, and your right hand from the groin crease toward your outer hip. This conscious touch gives your hip and thigh a sense of direction, supporting external rotation of the femur while releasing the hip bone. Breathe in and out. Come out of the pose. Repeat these actions on the other side.

Notice how your sacrum feels and whether this is an effective adjustment for you. Do not repeat it if it does not feel beneficial.

9. HALF MOON POSE (ARDHA CHANDRASANA)

Half Moon Pose is a strong hip-opening pose and thus can be very beneficial for relieving jaw tension thanks to the core link. It requires balance, so take care getting into and coming out of this pose. You should feel at ease holding Warrior 2 and Side Angle poses before attempting Half Moon. We'll practice a variation with your back to the wall for support. If you have a corner wall available where one side is as long as you are tall, this is especially effective for opening the hips. A variation where just the foot is at the wall with your back away from the wall follows in the notes for this pose. This is helpful if you have more stability and perhaps a little less wall space.

Props needed: Yoga mat, 2 blocks

Setup: It's important that the heel of your standing leg be a leg's length away from the wall. You can measure this by sitting on the floor, legs extended, with your feet to the wall. Place a block next to your hips. The block marks where the foot of your standing leg will go. Then, stand in Wide Leg Pose with the outside of your left foot at the wall and your right foot where your block indicates and your back to the adjacent wall. This will be a slightly shorter stance that usual for Wide Leg Pose.

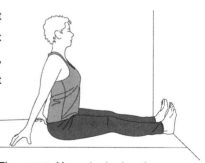

Figure 11.12: Measuring leg length.

Bring your right foot (standing leg) a few inches out from the wall at your back. This will leave room for your hips once your left leg is lifted. Bend your knee as you reach your right hand to the floor or block on your standing-leg side. Then raise your left leg, bringing the back of your leg to the wall behind you and the sole of your foot on the adjacent wall of your corner. Once you're in the pose, rest your back against the wall. Extend your arms, resting them against the wall, with palms facing forward.

Keep your gaze forward. Do not turn your head in this pose. Keep your arms and legs active, even while you have the support of the wall. Broaden your shoulders against the wall, engaging shoulder core actions and opening your chest. The back of your head can rest against the wall. Hold here for three to five breaths initially, staying longer as you are more at ease.

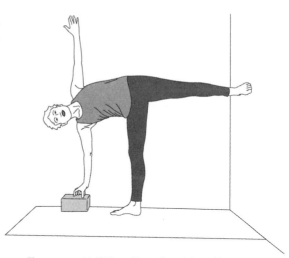

Figure 11.13: Half-Moon Pose. Practicing with your back to the wall is stabilizing and supports hip opening.

ARMS AND SHOULDERS—CORE ACTION 2 (PAGE 124)

Once you feel stable, extend both arms straight out from your shoulders. Your right hand will be on the floor or a block (or two—create a block tower if you need more height). Your left arm extends toward the ceiling. Lift your sternum and release your shoulder blades away from your ears. Broaden across the upper back and chest. Remember the shoulder blade actions: shoulders release down your back as the shoulder blades move away from each other and connect to the ribs at the back of your body. If you're one of those with more flexibility, try expanding the ribs of your upper back to connect with the scapulae. Stretch through your fingertips.

▣ HEAD AND TORSO

Do not turn your head. This pose is often taught with the head turned to look toward the ceiling; however, for our work with jaw tension it is important to keep your head and neck in a neutral position. As your shoulders open and stabilize, notice the curves of your spine. Lengthen your neck, extending through the top of your head.

▣ JAW—CORE ACTION 1 (PAGE 122)

Exhaling, open your mouth and extend your tongue in Lion Face Pose. Allow your jaw to relax. Notice the effect on your TMJs. Can you feel the difference between the right and left TMJs? Which side feels more open and which feels tighter?

To come out, exhale and bend your right knee and lower your left foot down to the floor at the wall, with a straight leg. Inhale as you straighten your right leg and stand up. Turn your feet to face forward. Step your feet together. Release your arms to your sides. Stand and breathe in Mountain Pose. Repeat on the other side.

Note: In this pose the right and left legs are doing very different things. The standing leg is strongly externally rotated. The elevated leg is in neutral rotation. The strength of the elevated leg can lessen the load on the standing leg, bringing a lightness to the pose and facilitating hip opening. To access this, press the foot of your elevated leg firmly against the wall as though you were standing on the floor. Then invite the pelvis to lift off of the femur of the standing leg.

Be aware of the standing-leg hip—you don't want it to rise, shortening your waist, which is likely to happen if the hip is tight. Encourage the standing-leg front hip bone to drop slightly and the elevated-leg hip bone to lift gently, with the intention to balance your pelvis.

Take note of the sacrum and sacroiliac joints, as well as how the femurs rest in the hip sockets. Does the weight-bearing leg feel jammed? Is there compression on either side? Working with the rotation of the legs and release of the pelvis can bring relief.

This is also an excellent pose for work with the feet. Remember the three lines defining your arches. Bring your mind to your feet and notice what areas are having difficulty working. See if you can feel both feet working equally despite the differences in the weight and positions.

If you have the stability, you might try practicing this pose with your back away from the wall and just the sole of your foot at the wall. It requires more balance, and you get a bit less information from the wall. However, it can also be a powerful hip-opening pose.

Place your mat with the short end at the wall. Measure leg length as above. Then stand in Wide Leg Pose with the outside of your left foot at the wall. Point your left toes thirty degrees away from the wall, rotating your left femur slightly in. Turn your right leg out ninety degrees, rotating from the top of your right femur. Bend your right knee and place your right hand on the floor or on a block (or two) outside of and a couple inches forward of your foot. Inhaling, lift your left leg up, keeping it straight. Straighten your right leg and place your left foot on the wall at hip height. Come out as described above.

10. WIDE LEG POSE FORWARD BEND (ADHO MUKHA PADOTTANASANA)

Let's revisit Wide Leg Pose, this time with forward bending. We have experienced how beneficial forward bending can be for working with jaw tension in Downward Dog Pose. There is a similar benefit here, with the addition of the hip opening that this pose offers. In this pose the weight stays on your legs. For many this allows for a greater range of motion in the shoulders. As a result, it's easier to engage the shoulder actions. Forward bending with the shoulders engaged can provide passive traction to the head, neck, and jaw. This is helpful in our work with jaw tension. We will practice forward bending in Wide Leg Pose as a progression through two different stages, moving from spinal extension to flexion. If you feel tired, take a break between these stages.

Props needed: Yoga mat
Optional props: 2 blocks or a chair

Standing on your yoga mat, begin in Mountain Pose (figure 11.7). Exhaling, separate your feet four to four and a half feet apart to Wide Leg Pose (figure 11.8). Place your hands at the groin crease where your thighs join your hips. Spread your toes wide. Inhaling, press down through your outer feet while lifting at the inner arches. Try to keep the entire line of your outer feet in contact with the floor. On your next breath, as you press down through your feet, feel your body lengthen upward through the top of your head.

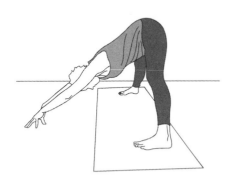

Figure 11.14: Wide Leg Pose Forward Bend, stage 1—extended spine. Place your hands at an appropriate height to allow your back to extend. You can use blocks on the low or high side, a chair seat, or a countertop as needed.

Exhaling, bend forward from your hips with your torso and head extended, chest open. Imagine releasing the tops of your femurs and inner groin backward (a slight internal rotation of femurs) as you extend your torso forward and lift the back of your hips up (untucking your pelvis). Now straighten your arms, bringing your hands to the floor. If it's difficult to reach the floor, use a block under each hand or place your hands on a firm chair seat. Lowering your torso, reach your arms forward as in Downward Dog Pose. If you are using blocks or a chair, slide them forward as needed. Keep your hips directly above your heels. Your legs are in Wide Leg Pose and your torso in Downward Dog. Stay for three to five breaths in each stage initially, and longer as you feel more at ease in the pose.

■ Shoulder Blades—Core Action 2 (page 124)

Apply the core actions for your shoulders: releasing your shoulder blades down your back toward your hips, broadening your upper back and chest, and connecting to your back ribs. When connecting, be careful not to overly press your shoulder blades down toward the ground but rather engage your shoulder blades while keeping the sternum lifted and open. Remember: the ribs at the back of your body may need to expand to support the connection with your shoulder blades.

■ Hips: Femur Rotation—Core Action 3 (page 133)

Notice the heads of your thighbones and how they rest into your pelvis. How does your sacrum feel? Bending your knees slightly, very gently experiment with internally and externally rotating your thighbones. Notice your breath and the quality of feeling in your abdomen and pelvis. Which rotation has the greatest sense of opening and connection? Restraighten your legs and see how the subtle rotation of the thighbones impacts you. Can you soften and use a little less effort? This will allow energy to move more freely through your body.

■ JAW—CORE ACTION 1 (PAGE 122)

Exhaling, open your mouth and face, extending your tongue in Lion Face Pose. Inhale through your nose, close your mouth while keeping space between your upper and lower teeth. Do not allow your upper and lower teeth to touch. Open and close three to five times. How does your jaw feel? Pay attention to the right and left sides and any connections you feel between your jaw, neck, shoulders, pelvis, and feet.

Caution: If your hands are on a chair, do not attempt stage 2; instead, skip ahead for instructions on how to come out of this pose.

■ STAGE 2: HANDS BETWEEN YOUR FEET

Exhaling, slide your hands—with your blocks, if you are using them—backward between your feet, bringing your fingertips in line with your toes with your palms on the floor, fingers extended. Bend your elbows, allowing your back to round slightly as your torso and head release toward the floor. Keep your elbows shoulder-width apart. If your head rests on the floor easily, then bring your feet a little closer together so that it is not touching.

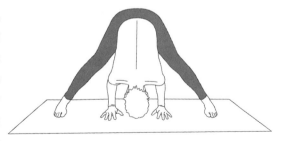

Figure 11.15: Wide Leg Pose Forward Bend, spinal flexion—shoulders relaxed. Place your hands at an appropriate height to support accessing the shoulder action

■ SHOULDER BLADES—CORE ACTION 2 (PAGE 124)

Initially allow your shoulder blades to relax toward your head and the floor. Then, keeping your elbows bent, inhale and draw your shoulder blades up your back, toward your hips. Try to isolate the action of your shoulder blades. Relax and engage several times, refining your effort. There should be minimal movement in your back, spine, and head when engaging the scapulae. For example, if

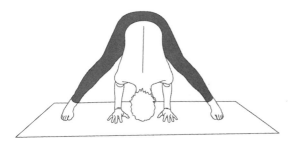

Figure 11.16: Wide Leg Pose Forward Bend, spinal flexion—shoulders engaged. Place your hands at an appropriate height to support accessing the shoulder action

your back begins to extend or arch, this is too much movement. Likewise your head should not lift. Activating the shoulder blades correctly stabilizes C7 (the seventh cervical vertebra—the base of your neck), which in turn allows the neck and head to hang more freely, receiving passive traction in the inverted pose. Once you are able to access released scapulae—which is actually elevating them because you are inverted—then apply the broadening and connecting actions.

▪ HIPS—CORE ACTION 3 (PAGE 133)

Reconnect to the heads of your thighbones where they rest into your hips. Bending your knees slightly, experiment with gentle internal and external rotation. Notice your breath and the quality of feeling in your abdomen and pelvis. Restraighten your legs and try again. Which rotation allows for the greatest sense of opening and connection?

▪ JAW—CORE ACTION 1 (PAGE 122)

Exhaling, open your mouth and face, extending your tongue in Lion Face Pose. Inhaling through your nose, close your mouth without allowing your upper and lower teeth to touch. Open and close three to five times. How does your jaw feel as you repeat this pose? Pay attention to your right and left sides and any connections you feel between your jaw, neck, shoulders, pelvis, and feet.

To come out: First bring your hands to your hips, where your thighs join your pelvis. Inhaling, extend your torso forward and rise up to standing. Exhaling, step your feet together. Release your arms and stand in Mountain Pose.

Modification: If your back is weak or vulnerable, you can practice with your torso resting on a table, countertop, or the back of a chair—anything stable that is about the same height as your hips or slightly higher. In this case you would enter the pose differently:

Stand in front of the table or countertop in Wide Leg Pose. Exhaling, place your hands on the table. Inhaling, lengthen upward from your feet through the top of your head. Exhaling, bend your knees slightly and gently lower your torso to rest on the table, using your hands for support. Experiment with engaging the core actions as above.

11. Bridge Pose (Setu Bandha Sarvangasana)

Chronic jaw tension can lead to tight shoulders and a contracted chest. Bridge Pose is great for opening these areas as well as strengthening your back. A preparation is provided that will likely be accessible to most everyone. It offers an exploration of the spinal curves, as well as the rotation of humeri and femurs, providing tactile information about how your hips, back, chest, neck, and jaw are connected. Go slow and repeat this several times to allow your body and mind to fully absorb the experience.

The full version provided here was affectionately dubbed "Our Favorite Bridge Pose" by author and yoga teacher Donald Moyer. The nickname provided a cue for us to collect our props—which gives you an idea why other teachers have called it "Supported Bridge." I find this setup particularly good for working with jaw tension for a few reasons. Blankets support your shoulders and help protect the natural curve of your neck. The height under your hips provides a lovely opening to the chest. Higher is more beneficial, provided you have the flexibility. It will reduce the weight on your shoulders, allowing your chest to open more fully. In order to practice the complete pose, your lower back and hips will need to have some amount of strength and flexibility.

Caution: Do not practice Lion Face in this pose. Your head is fixed against the floor and thus cannot release backward. Opening your mouth wide may result in neck discomfort. Do not turn your head once your hips are lifted in the full pose. This can result in neck strain. The full pose is not recommended during menstruation.

Props needed: Yoga mat (optional)

Lie down on your back, with your knees bent and the soles of your feet on the mat, as close as possible to your buttocks. Have your arms at your sides, palms down. Feel your lower back on the floor. Exhaling, drop your chin down toward your chest (without lifting your head).

Inhaling, externally rotate your shoulders, allowing your arms and palms to turn up while lifting your sternum toward your chin. Allow your chin to lift

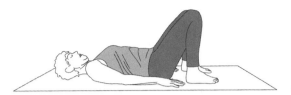

Figure 11.17: Bridge Pose prep, stage 1—exhale. Palms down, shoulders rolled forward, low back resting on floor (flattened lumbar and cervical curve); chest and chin dropped.

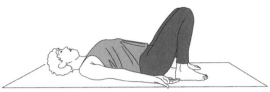

Figure 11.18: Bridge Pose prep, stage 2—inhale. Palms up, shoulders to the floor, chest and chin lifted, and natural lumbar (lordosis) and cervical curves.

slightly in response to the sternum lift. Press your shoulder blades onto the floor. Broaden your upper back and chest. Connect the scapulae and back ribs. Remember your core action for the shoulders: release, broaden, connect.

Bring attention to your hips. Allow your lumbar curve (lordosis) to increase, tilting your pelvis slightly and opening your chest. To clarify this, imagine a clock dial on your sacrum, with 12 o'clock at the top near your lumbar and 6 o'clock at your tailbone. Tilt your pelvis from 12 to 6. Exhaling, return to the initial position with palms down. Repeat three to five times, in coordination with your breathing.

"OUR FAVORITE BRIDGE POSE"

Props needed: Yoga mat, thick block, skinny block, 1 or 2 blankets folded narrow, yoga strap

Setup: Place a folded blanket across your mat, one-third of the way from the end. Have the other props within reach. Buckle the strap, creating a loop that's a little wider than shoulder width.

Lie down with your shoulders resting on the blanket. Place the top of your shoulders just below the blanket's folded edge. Your head and neck will be on your mat above the blanket. Bend your knees, bringing your feet on the mat, close to your hips. Inhaling, lift your hips and place a thick block widthwise under your hips at the highest comfortable height. (Those with greater flexibility can use two blocks, with the skinny block on the low side providing a pedestal.) Lower your sacrum to rest on the block. Lift your chest and shoulders so that you are resting on the tops of the shoulders. Arms are

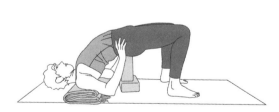

Figure 11.19: Our Favorite Bridge Pose. Place the props carefully before doing the pose.

at your sides, palms up. Stay here for three to five breaths initially, lengthening your time in the pose as you feel more at ease.

▦ SHOULDERS—CORE ACTION 2 (PAGE 124)

As you rest on the block with your hips lifted, your scapulae should be off the floor, releasing away from your ears. Lift your sternum, broadening your chest and upper back. Practice the shoulder core action: Connect your shoulder blades to your upper ribs at the back of your body. Breathe into your upper back to invite your ribs to connect with your shoulder blades. Soften your abdomen.

With micromovements, lift your sternum toward your chin, and then as you reengage the three-part shoulder action, very gently lift your chin toward the ceiling. Repeat this three or four times. These small, subtle movements can invite release of the upper cervical vertebrae and restore the upper cervical curve.

To come out: Inhaling, lift your hips up off the block. Use one hand to remove the block from under you. Keep your hips lifted. Now raise your arms toward the ceiling. Exhaling and rounding your back, lower your hips and back to the floor. Breathe and rest.

Inversions

Once we feel confidence and stability in standing poses, forward bends, and Downward Dog Pose, we can begin to explore inverting. Adho Mukha Svanasana serves as a gateway to the inverted poses. It offers us the opportunity to develop the strength, stability, and flexibility needed for full inversions. It's very important to be patient and take the time to feel at ease in Downward Dog and Wide Leg Pose Forward Bend before attempting more challenging poses. When inverting, we face the issue of disorientation. Up becomes down, and down becomes up. How do we work in the pose?! For most, the excitement of inverting makes it difficult to apply awareness in the pose initially. If you are still exploring how to invert, becoming oriented in a disorienting situation, and working with the thrill and excitement of turning the world upside down, then inversions will not be helpful for jaw tension (though they may be a lot of fun and beneficial in other ways!).

Some inversions have a role to play in our journey to heal jaw tension, but only if we know how to work effectively in the poses. The inverted poses included here are intended for experienced practitioners. For those who are new to yoga, seek the guidance of a skilled teacher to learn how to practice safely before attempting inversions on your own.

For relief from jaw tension, head and neck compressive inversions such as head balance and shoulder balance are not recommended due to the connection between the jaw and neck. Inversions where the head can hang freely can be beneficial—if we are able to engage the shoulders and keep the head and neck passive. This action is explored in detail in Wide Leg Pose Forward Bend with spinal flexion (page 161). Becoming familiar with this before attempting other inversions in this program will facilitate your experience and make it more beneficial.

Inversions should not be practiced if you are having a migraine or other headache, or during menstruation. More information on inversions is provided in the chapter 12 Yoga Practice Sequences.

12. HALF HANDSTAND

This pose is sometimes called L Pose or Reverse Tabletop Pose. As we experienced in Downward Dog Pose, going upside down can be very beneficial for relieving jaw tension. Half Handstand can likewise be a supportive pose for working with jaw tension—once we are able to access the shoulder actions regularly in Downward Dog. Half Handstand requires more strength and stability than Downward Dog, but it may be more accessible to some than Full Handstand or Elbow Balance. For working with jaw tension, I recommend using a strap at your elbows to help stabilize your arms. This will make it easier to access the shoulder actions and is helpful both for hypermobility (because it protects the elbow joints) and/or tight shoulders (because the increased stability will help you to work more effectively). Additionally, a lift under the palms can reduce strain on the wrists. This optional support will be described after the main pose.

Caution: It is important to keep your head and neck passive in this pose. Do not lift your head. Inverting is not recommended during menstruation, as it interferes with the natural downward flow occurring.

Props needed: Wall

Optional props: 1 or 2 yoga mats, block, yoga strap

Setup: It is important that your hands be placed a little more than a leg's length from the wall. To measure this, sit down with your legs extended and your heels at the wall. Place a block next to your outer hip. The block marks where your hands will go. (See figure 11.12 on page 157.) Now make a loop in your yoga strap and place it around your upper arms. Adjust the strap to hold your arms shoulder-width apart. To stabilize your elbows, place the strap directly over the elbow joints. To stabilize your arms and shoulders, try placing your strap just above your elbows, on your upper arms. Once you are in the pose, let your forehead rest against the strap.

To go into the pose, kneel on your mat with your feet touching the wall and the strap around your arms. Place your hands shoulder-width apart on your mat, in line with your block. Exhaling, lift your hips to a modified Downward Dog with your heels at the wall.

Keeping your arms straight without hyperextending your elbows, walk your feet up the wall until they are level with your hips. Keep your head and neck passive. Press your feet—especially your heels—against the wall to stabilize yourself. Stay here for three to five breaths initially, then longer as the pose becomes easier.

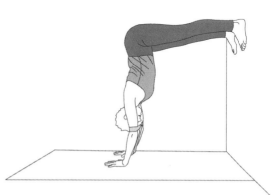

Figure 11.20: Half Handstand with strap. The strap at or just above elbows helps to engage your shoulders and avoid hyperextension. Moving your hands an extra inch or two away from the wall will help with balancing.

SHOULDERS—CORE ACTION 2: RELEASE, BROADEN, CONNECT (PAGE 124)

When you are upside down, *releasing* your shoulder blades becomes *lifting* them up your back toward your hips. Otherwise, the action is the same as previously. Bending your knees slightly can help stabilize your pose as you broaden your upper back and chest, as well as your shoulder blades against the ribs at the back of your body. Experiment with pressing your shoulder blades onto your ribs versus expanding your upper back ribs into your shoulder blades, especially if you have loose or hypermobile joints. Activating your shoulders and arms can help to lighten the pose.

▦ Hips—Core Action 3 (page 133)

With straight arms and engaged shoulders, see if you can create some space in your torso and hips. With knees slightly bent, imagine your ribs lifting off of your shoulders, your hips lifting away from your ribs, and your thighbones off of your pelvis. Take the backs of your thighs toward the ceiling. Invite a subtle rotation of the femur heads in the hip sockets.

▦ Jaw—Core Action 1 (page 122)

Slowly open and close your mouth gently three to five times in Lion Face Pose. There is no need to open wide or extend your tongue while inverted. We're more focused on small movements and microadjustments. Because you are inverted your shoulders are working harder, which will have a noticeable impact on the TMJs. Opening your mouth may feel quite different than when standing upright. Right-left tension patterns can be more apparent, which can be a super beneficial experience to learn from. As much as possible, relax your jaw, and pay close attention to how your TMJs respond.

To come out: Exhaling, bring one foot at a time back to the floor near the wall. Bend your knees and rest in Child's Pose.

Modification: lift beneath hands to decrease wrist strain—fold a yoga mat in half three times. Place your palms on the folded mat with your knuckles just at the edge of it and your fingers on the floor. Extend your fingers and hands. The yoga mat acts as a lift, taking some of the weight off of the wrists in this pose. A yoga wedge with a mat over it can also serve this purpose.

13. Handstand (Adho Mukha Vrksasana)

Handstands can be a great asset in our work with jaw tension—provided you have the strength, flexibility, and skill to perform this pose. When we go upside down, we are reversing the effects of gravity. That means you can decompress parts of your body that have been under pressure over the years from this constant force. It's important that the shoulders work correctly in this pose. When we engage the shoulders upside down, this stabilizes the seventh cervical vertebra, which allows the neck and head—including the jaw—to receive passive traction. This can be very beneficial for relieving jaw tension. Downward Dog Pose gives us a taste of this. Practicing Downward Dog regularly over time can help to prepare your body for Handstand.

We'll practice a variation at the wall, with the head and neck released, as well as support at the elbows. Optional wrist support is described below as a modification.

Caution: Do not lift your head in this pose. It is important when working with jaw tension to keep the head and neck passive. This is due to the connection between the jaw, neck, and shoulders. When opening your mouth in this pose, go slowly and gently. Inverting during menstruation is not recommended.

Props needed: Wall

Optional props: 1 or 2 yoga mats, strap with buckle

Place a buckled yoga strap around your elbows. Adjust the buckle to hold your arms shoulder-width apart. Make sure the buckle is in the space between your arms, where it cannot pinch your skin. Stretch your arms out in front of you while pressing into the strap. Your hands should be shoulder-width apart. Place your hands on the floor while pressing into the strap. Once you are in the pose, let your head rest on the strap.

Now kneel on the floor with your fingertips about six inches from the wall. Press your fingers into the floor and bring a lightness to your palms. Try to have your fingers feel stronger and more stable than the palms of your hands; this will help you lift out of your wrists.

Raise your hips into a modified (shorter) Downward Dog Pose. Walk one foot in, bending the knee. Keeping the other leg straight, swing your legs up into a Handstand. Let the bent leg follow the momentum of the straight leg. Straighten your second leg out quickly. It's important to keep both arms and legs straight once your feet have left the floor; otherwise, you'll lose momentum. Bring your heels to the wall with your feet flexed. Keep your head and neck passive.

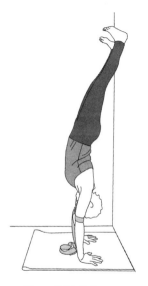

Figure 11.21: Full arm balance at wall with elbow strap. The strap at or just above elbows helps to engage your shoulders and avoid hyperextension of the elbow joint.

ARMS AND SHOULDERS—CORE ACTION 2 (PAGE 124)

Since you are upside down, releasing your shoulder blades becomes lifting them up your back toward your hips. The action is the same as earlier. Broaden your upper back and chest. Connect your shoulder blades to the ribs at the back of your body. Stay here for three to five breaths initially, and then longer as you feel more at ease.

◼ HIPS—CORE ACTION 3 (PAGE 133)

Once you feel stable in the pose, imagine lifting your rib cage off of your shoulders, then lifting your pelvis off of your rib cage, and then lifting your thighbones off of your pelvis. As you create more space in your hips, allow your femurs to gently rotate internally, broadening your sacrum between the pelvic bones. Lift your tail to lengthen your lower back.

◼ JAW—CORE ACTION 1 (PAGE 122)

Gently open and close your mouth three to five times in Lion Face Pose while in Handstand. There's no need to open wide or extend your tongue. Instead, focus on micromovements. Since your shoulders are working hard to hold you up, this will have an impact on your TMJs. There may be less range of motion in your mouth. Notice the effects of opening and closing on your jaw and neck. Right-left imbalances may well be more dramatic while inverted. This is a lot of information to absorb while inverted. Go slow and pay attention.

To come out: Exhaling and keeping your arms and legs straight, extend one leg at a time to the floor. Then bend your knees and rest in Child's Pose.

Modifications: Wrist support—if your wrists feel uncomfortable, you can try this approach. Fold your yoga mat in half three times. Place your folded mat parallel to the wall, six to nine inches away. Place your palms on your mat with your fingers off the mat and pointing toward the wall. Your knuckles are just at the edge of the mat. Extend your fingers and hands.

Shoulder blade support—If you find it difficult to access your shoulder core actions, this approach encourages the external rotation of your upper arms, which will help stabilize your shoulder blades against your upper back. Fold your yoga mat in half three times. Place your mat on the floor about six inches from the wall. Turning your hands away from each other, place your palms on the outer edges of your mat. Your arms are externally rotated. Your fingertips are facing away from each other. Your palms are on your mat, knuckles at the edge, and fingertips on the floor. For extra stability, add a strap at your elbows.

Note: When you open and close your mouth during Handstand, the force of gravity and extra effort of your shoulders due to holding up your body weight increase pressure on the TMJs. You may feel the imbalance of your TMJs more clearly. Keeping your head and neck passive allows your neck, and particularly the cervical spine, to decompress. Think of your head as a bowling ball, just hanging, suspended from the rope of your spine. As you now know, your TMJs, head, neck, and shoulders are intertwined. If you have the strength and flexibility to access Handstand, it can be very beneficial in your work with jaw tension.

14. Elbow Balance (Pincha Mayurasana)

Elbow Balance is an excellent pose for working with jaw tension if you have enough strength and stability. Interestingly, if you are comfortable in this pose, you may find it easier to access the shoulder core action in Elbow Balance than Handstand.

For our purpose of working with jaw tension we will practice a variation near the wall with a few props for support. Think of how your feet work in Mountain Pose. In Elbow Balance, your forearms become your feet. Your hands and fingers are your toes, and your elbows are your heels. It is important that your elbows, forearms, hands, and fingers provide a stable base of support for your body when you take the full pose. Notice the tendency for hands and wrists to lift and rotate. Try to keep an even contact and length from elbow to fingertips when in this pose. If you have difficulty keeping your forearms lengthened on the floor, try the variation with your palms facing the blocks.

Caution: Do not lift your head in this pose. Keep your head and neck released. Your head should not touch the floor at any time in this pose, including when going in and out. Inverting during menstruation is not recommended.

Props needed: Yoga mat, blanket, strap, 1 or 2 blocks, wall
Optional props: Blanket

Setup: Fold the yoga mat in half twice, and place it at the wall. The mat will cushion your elbows and forearms. If you want extra padding, add a firm folded blanket on top. Make a loop in your strap and put it around your arms, just above your elbows. Adjust the strap to hold your elbows shoulder-width apart. (Check this

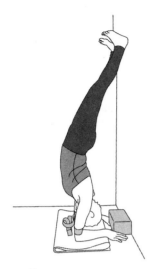

Figure 11.22:
Elbow Balance at
wall with elbow
strap.

by extending your arms with palms facing each other while pressing into the strap. Your hands should remain in line with your shoulders.)

Bring your forearms to your mat, with hands on either side of your block, palms down and fingers extended. Your thumbs and index fingers will cradle the lower corners of the block. Bring the whole forearm into contact with the mat. Press down at the inner wrist, thumb, and index finger. Don't let these areas lift up. Lift your hips into a modified (shortened) Downward Dog Pose. Take a moment to feel the pressure of the forearms and wrists on your mat. Notice if portions have lifted, and press them back down onto your mat.

Once your forearms are well placed, firm the outer arms toward the inner arms so that you are no longer pressing into the strap. Lift and engage your shoulders, releasing your head and neck. Your head should hang freely but not touch the floor. Gently lift your legs or kick them up one at a time. Do not allow your head to sink down or rest on the floor when lifting your legs. Keep the shoulder blades engaged for strength. Initially bring your heels to rest against the wall with feet flexed—once you have strength and experience, you can have your heels in line with the rest of your body. Stay here for three to five breaths initially, and then longer as you feel more at ease.

Now that you're in the full pose, reevaluate the contact and placement of your elbows, forearms, wrists, hands, and fingers. Balance the pressure between your inner and outer arms and your right and left sides. Strengthen and lengthen. Straighten your fingers. Lift out of your thumbs and bring more weight to your other fingers.

■ **SHOULDERS—CORE ACTION 2 (PAGE 124)**

Since you are inverted, releasing your shoulder blades becomes lifting them up toward your hips. Broaden your upper back and chest. Connect your shoulder blades and ribs at the back of your body by either pressing your shoulder blades onto your back or expanding your back ribs toward your shoulder blades. Lift your ribs off of your shoulders. Keep your head and neck passive. Your head should not touch the floor. Engaging your shoulder blades will keep your head off the floor.

PELVIS AND LEGS—CORE ACTION 3 (PAGE 133)

Bring your hips over your torso, and imagine lifting your pelvis off your ribs. Lengthen your legs up out of the hips, taking the soles of your feet toward the ceiling. Keep your feet flexed, as though standing on the ceiling. Notice how your sacrum feels. Is it compressed? Experiment with a slight internal rotation to the thighbones to help broaden and free your sacrum. Lift your tail to lengthen your lower back.

JAW—CORE ACTION 1 (PAGE 122)

With your shoulders, hips, and feet engaged, open and close your mouth three to five times in Lion Face Pose. As in the other inversions, there's no need to open wide or extend your tongue. Focus on gentle micromovements. See if you can notice how this impacts your TMJs. Opening and closing your mouth while inverted with shoulders engaged can facilitate decompressing the TMJs and the upper cervical spine. You may experience a smaller range of motion. The right-left imbalances may be more apparent. Go slow and pay close attention to your experience.

To come out, keep your shoulders engaged. Exhaling, lower your legs gently one at a time to the floor, returning to Downward Dog Pose. Stay here for a couple of breaths. Bend your knees and rest in Child's Pose.

Modification: If it is very difficult to keep the inner wrist down, try placing your palms against the sides of the block. Keep all fingers extended, with pinkie fingers, outer wrists, and forearms in a straight line and in contact with the floor. Try not to have any gaps between the floor and your forearms, wrists, and pinkie fingers at any point in this pose.

Note: Elbow Balance is for intermediate and advanced yoga practitioners. Do not attempt this pose if you are not comfortable with inverting, balancing, and/or lack arm strength. Downward Dog Pose and Wide Leg Pose Forward Bend can provide similar benefit.

Corpse Pose (Savasana)

The final pose in any yoga sequence is Savasana. This is where we receive the benefit of our entire practice. Translated as "Corpse Pose," Savasana is a time of stillness and rest. While the association with corpses may initially be unappealing, it can also be viewed in a positive light. Corpses are calm, peaceful, at ease. They have relinquished the struggles of daily life. And they are very, very quiet. These are the qualities we can aspire to in this practice.

Whatever you do, do not skip this pose. Even if you only practice one or two poses, take a bit of time to rest in Savasana before going on with your day. In the Jaw Tension Explained section, we explored the relationship between your nervous system and jaw tension. The more active yoga poses help to spread mindful awareness throughout your body, integrating awareness and increasing parasympathetic activity while decreasing sympathetic activity. With Corpse Pose we are deepening the experience of relaxation, inviting a pleasant state of rest and renewal. This is a time for body and mind to integrate the efforts applied during your asana practice.

Two variations are offered here. Reclining Bound Angle Pose is excellent for opening the hips and chest, which is not only restorative but also will improve breathing. As we have noted, breathing is often restricted from jaw tension. Thus this pose is an excellent remedy for clenchers and grinders.

Traditional Corpse Pose is a simple option, accessible to almost everyone. Three-Part Breathing (page 212) is recommended as a way to begin this pose (once you are settled into it). And then stay . . . for anywhere from 5–20 minutes, or longer. Consider following this practice with a guided meditation from part three, Mindfulness Exercises. Audio recordings of guided meditations are available for free download at www.catorshachoy.com.

15. RECLINING BOUND ANGLE POSE (SUPTA BADDHA KONASANA)

Reclining Bound Angle Pose is deeply relaxing and comforting. The use of props is designed to help your body to be fully at ease in this pose. You are not looking for a strong stretch but rather to feel so entirely supported that you let go of effort and truly rest. This pose encourages a passive opening of the belly, hips, and chest—particularly when the bolster (or folded blankets) is slightly narrower than your torso. Blankets are used to fully support your shoulders, neck, and head. There should be contact under the length of your spine. Once in the pose, we will practice Three-Part Breathing (page 212) to foster breath awareness and relaxation. This is an excellent way to reset your nervous system.

Caution: Unsupported limbs can potentially overstretch joints and cause lasting damage. Take time to set this pose up carefully. Supported limbs create safety, allowing your nervous system to settle. In this way you will receive the most benefit.

Props needed: Yoga mat, 2–4 yoga blankets, 2 blocks, bolster
(1 or 2 blankets can be substituted for a bolster)
Optional props: hand towel, additional yoga blankets or towels.
You may want to place a blanket lengthwise over your yoga mat for additional cushion if the floor is hard.

Setup: Position your bolster lengthwise, at one end of your mat. Center it width-wise. Fold a blanket in half and place it so that it covers the top two-thirds of your bolster. This will support your shoulders. Fold a second blanket in thirds and put it on top of the first blanket, covering the top third of the bolster. This will create a pillow for your head and neck. Put blocks on either side of the yoga mat, below the bolster.

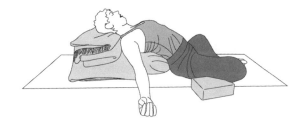

Figure 11.23:
Reclining Bound Angle Pose.

Sit on the floor with your sacrum touching the narrow end of your bolster and your legs extended in front of you. Bend your knees, placing your feet on the floor. Put your hands behind you on your bolster, as you lower your back down onto it. Once you are lying down comfortably, open your knees out to the sides, bringing the soles of your feet together. Move blocks under your thighs to allevi-ate any strain. Rest your arms on the floor in a relaxed way, palms up. If your arms do not easily reach the floor, use additional folded blankets or towels underneath them. Stay here for five minutes or longer, based on your level of comfort.

Once you are settled into Reclining Bound Angle Pose, practice Three-Part Breathing. See instructions on page 212.

To come out: Exhaling, straighten your legs on the floor, flexing your feet. Stay here for a couple of breaths. Then, as you exhale, bend your right knee and place your foot on the floor near your hips. Breathe in. Exhaling, repeat this move with the left leg. On the next exhale turn to rest on your right side on the floor, gently sliding off your bolster. Exhaling, use your left hand on the floor in front of you to push yourself up to sitting.

Troubleshooting: If your back is uncomfortable, it may help to move your hips an inch or two away from the bolster. You can also try raising or lowering the height of the bolster by adding a folded blanket lengthwise under it or using one or two blankets folded lengthwise instead of the bolster.

To ease discomfort in the hips or sacroiliac joints, try adjusting the height of the blocks under your thighs. Folded blankets or towels can be used instead of blocks. It is important to support your thighs even if you have the flexibility to rest your legs on the floor. Staying in this pose is not about feeling a strong stretch in your muscles but rather letting your abdomen relax, your chest open, and your body feel supported.

The curve of your neck should be fully supported in this reclining pose. Adjust the blankets as needed. You can also use a rolled-up hand towel or washcloth for neck support. If the support is not comfortable, remove or change it.

16. Traditional Corpse Pose (Savasana)

This pose is a simple set-up on the floor. It can also be done on a bed or sofa, provided there is space to place your body carefully in a balanced way.

Props needed: Yoga mat, 2–4 blankets, bolster or pillow (or folded blankets)
Optional props: rolled-up hand towel for under your neck

Setup: Place your yoga mat on the floor with enough space around it so you are not immediately touching any walls or furniture. If the floor is hard or cold, you may want to place a blanket on top of the mat. Place a folded blanket at one end of your mat for your head. Place a bolster or two blankets, folded long and narrow, a little below the middle of your mat—this will support your knees. You may wish to have a blanket over you for comfort.

Lie down on your side with knees bent, just to the side of your mat with your

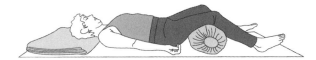

Figure 11.24. Savasana.

head on the blanket. Exhaling, roll onto your back. Allow your legs to extend over the bolster or folded blankets. Adjust your body so that it is balanced, with your head centered on the blanket, shoulders on the mat, arms equi-distant from your sides, hips balanced, legs relaxed, knees supported, and feet a little wider than hip-distance apart. Ideally the bolster is placed under the lower thighs. Adjust the bolster so that it feels most supportive to your body, allowing your low back and hips to fully relax. Support the curve of your neck by rolling up the lower edge of the blanket under your head just the right amount or using a rolled hand towel. Once you find ease and balance in the posture, let your body become still. Practice Three-Part Breathing (page 212) and then stay as long as is comfortable. Consider following this with a guided meditation practice from part three, Mindfulness Exercises. Audio recordings are available for free download at www.catorshachoy.com.

Yoga Practice Sequences

Notes

PLEASE LISTEN to your body and respect your personal limitations. The poses presented are suggestions for personal practice. All poses may not be suitable for everyone. Please consult with your medical professional before beginning any physical practice to be sure it is suitable for you. Pay attention to your experience. If you are in pain or uncomfortable, come out of the pose immediately. Seek guidance from a qualified instructor before resuming practice.

If you are new to yoga, try holding a pose for three breaths—inhale and exhale slowly three times unless otherwise specified in the yoga pose instructions. Over time you can build up to thirty seconds for standing poses, and then one minute. Try to practice Savasana for a minimum of five minutes initially. Build up to fifteen or more minutes. Using a timer is helpful for relaxation poses.

If you have an established yoga practice, you can hold poses for longer if this is comfortable for you.

Inversions

Full inversions are included only in the full series of poses. I highly recommend receiving instruction from a qualified teacher before practicing inversions on your own. Inversions should not be practiced during migraines or sinus headaches or if you have high blood pressure, eye conditions, or a recent head or neck injury. Additionally, inverting during menstruation is not recommended as it interferes with the natural down and out flow.

For yogis who practice inversions regularly, I discourage practicing head-supported poses while attempting to relieve jaw tension. This includes a traditional form of head balance (Sirsasana) and shoulder balance (Sarvangasana). This is due to the connection between the jaw and the neck as described in part one (Guzay's theorem). Inversions where the head is free to hang can be beneficial for jaw tension if applied correctly. See chapter 11 for details.

The Basics: Foundational Practices

4 core actions: Use these exercises for accessing the actions for feet, hips, shoulders, and jaw (pages 122–42).

Limited Series—
Apply Foundational Actions in Each Pose

Standing Mountain Pose page 148 (11.7)

Cat/Dog Pose page 144 (11.1–11.3)

Puppy Pose page 145 (11.4)

Downward Dog Pose (Adho Mukha Svanasana) page 146 (11.6)

Child's Pose (Balasana) page 146 (11.5)

Wide Leg Pose (Padottanasana) page 149 (11.8)

Warrior 2 Pose (Virabhadrasana 2) page 153 (11.9)

Wide Leg Pose Forward Bend (Adho Mukha Padottanasana) page 160–62 (11.14–11.16)

Bridge Pose prep page 164 (11.17–11.18)

Savasana: Reclining Bound Angle Pose (Supta Baddha Konasana) page 175 (11.23) or 177 (11.24)

With Three-Part Breathing page 212

Followed by Breath Awareness page 216

(Audio downloads for breathing exercises are available at www.catorshachoy.com)

Extended Series: Emphasizes More Hip Opening

Add these standing poses after Warrior 2 Pose and before Wide Leg Pose Forward Bend:

Side Angle Pose (Parshva Konasana) page 155 (11.11)

Half Moon Pose (Ardha Chandrasana) page 157 (11.13)

Puppy Pose, Downward Dog Pose, Child's Pose (Adho Mukha Svanasana progression) page 146 (11.4–11.6)

Savasana: Reclining Bound Angle Pose (Supta Baddha Konasana) page 175 (11.23) or 177 (11.24)

With Three-Part Breathing page 212

Followed by Breath Awareness page 216

Full Series—For Intermediate Practitioners and Those with Full Range of Motion and Stability in Their Shoulders

Use the extended series above, and insert the following postures between Wide Leg Pose Forward Bend and Reclining Bound Angle Pose with Three-Part Breathing for Savasana.

Half Handstand page 167 (11.20)

Handstand (Adho Mukha Vrkhsasana) page 169 (11.21)

Elbow Balance (Pincha Mayurasana) page 172 (11.22)

Bridge Pose (Setu Bandha Sarvangasana) page 164 (11.19)

PART THREE

Mindfulness Exercises

⚘13

What Is Mindfulness?

Mindfulness means paying attention in a particular way: on purpose, in the present moment, and nonjudgmentally.

—JON KABAT-ZINN, FOUNDER OF THE MINDFULNESS-BASED
STRESS REDUCTION PROGRAM AT THE UNIVERSITY OF
MASSACHUSETTS MEDICAL CENTER

MINDFULNESS IS KNOWING what is happening *as it is happening*. It is the ability to consciously know our experience. We all have the capacity to be mindful. In fact, your mind is inherently aware and mindful. When we cultivate mindfulness, we are revealing the true nature of the mind— alert, curious, bright, aware, and present. You feel like this every day, right? (OK, so it may take a little practice . . . that's where this book comes in!)

There are moments in life when we are naturally mindful, when we are attuned to the subtleties of each moment. Our senses are heightened, everything seems new, bright, appearing in Technicolor, and it's as though time stands still—we lose a sense of time passing. These experiences of our natural awareness are sometimes called *beginner's mind*. This is because when we are new to something, often we have fewer concepts about it and are more able to simply be with the experience. We might liken this to how a young child is very much in the present moment and easily entertained. Having newly arrived on planet earth, they have fewer ideas about what *ought to* happen and so are frequently more accepting of things as they *are*. Have you ever watched a child play endlessly with a simple object? Or have you noticed them express repeated joy and laughter at the simplest of gestures you make, crying out, *again! again!* when your mind has long since moved on? The Zen master Shunryu Suzuki sums this up beautifully: *In the beginner's mind there are many possibilities, but in the expert's mind there are few.*

There are certain times when beginner's mind is likelier. For example, when you get unexpected news, a sudden surprise or shock can cause past and future to drop away instantly and heighten your senses. To this day there are many people who remember exactly where they were and what they were doing when they heard about the 9/11 attack on the World Trade Center in New York City in 2001. Similarly, friends who lived in California in 1989 recall with great clarity the experience of the Loma Prieta earthquake. But not all experiences of beginner's mind are associated with destructive events. What if you are seeing someone you love after a long separation? The intensity of your longing and anticipation falling away in the moment of actually being together again can bring you into the present moment very dramatically.

Your natural awareness might be revealed when biting into something you haven't eaten before and finding an unusual flavor hitting your taste buds. Yawning and laughing are often moments of spontaneous aware-ness. If you like competitive sports, the heightened awareness that results may well be a part of the appeal. Being *in the zone* (also called *flow state*) is a form of mindfulness. For many, exercising or dancing—doing focused, phys-ical movement—is a way to bring body and mind together, decrease think-ing, and arrive in the present moment. Training your mind on an activity is concentrating. Concentration makes the mind happy, relaxed, at ease. Being relaxed, at ease, and concentrated can facilitate the experience of the awake, aware nature of mind.

As an example, when I dive into water, I find myself immediately, natu-rally aware. It is such an exquisite experience that my senses are flooded with the unfolding of each moment. All thoughts disappear. My body moving through cool liquid water is so compelling, my attention does not wander. Past and future do not exist. The light shining through the water is incredi-bly beautiful. Holding my breath heightens the quiet of being underwater. I honestly forget about breathing for some period of time. Take a moment to reflect on when you have experienced beginner's mind. What occurs to you? Knowing your experiences of natural awareness can help you to understand mindfulness.

Mindfulness is not intellectual. It is that quality of mind that knows and records experience. Mindfulness comes through all the senses—seeing, hearing, touching, tasting, smelling—and thought. Knowing the texture of the chair you are sitting in, witnessing the quality of the light, hearing the sounds in your immediate environment, tasting the first bite of lunch. It is immediate, sensory, and impactful. It is not simply *noticing* these things; it is also *knowing* that you notice these things.

Mindfulness creates an opportunity to choose what to be aware of. There is so much happening in any given moment that our senses can easily become overwhelmed, leading us to shut down or zone out. But when we are mindful, we can decide where to apply our attention. This can help us to filter our experience and stay more present. In order to better understand how this works, let's conduct an experiment. Take a moment to sit and simply notice what you notice. After you finish reading this paragraph, sit quietly and pay attention to your experience for one minute. If you like, you can set a timer and use pen and paper to write it all down. Just find one word for each thing you notice in the next minute. It's fine if the same thing comes up more than once. Here's a hint: Observe the experience through each of your sense organs. Also, thoughts and emotions qualify as "things" on this list. Now settle your body. Take a conscious breath, and let it out. Are you ready to begin? Go!

So what did you notice?

You really can't do this wrong. Whatever you notice is exactly right. With regard to mindfulness, it doesn't really matter *what* your experience is. What matters is that you *know your experience.*

Watching the Movie of Life

Here's another way of understanding mindfulness. When we watch a movie, we tend to become absorbed in the story. We laugh when something funny happens; we cry when the story is sad; we feel afraid when it is scary or dramatic. However, if we are mindful, we recognize that these are actors performing a story. The story isn't real; it's a story. We can still enjoy the story, and laugh and cry, but we are less lost in the myth of it.

If we look even more closely we can realize that, actually, there aren't even actors; they performed the story in some other time and place. Right now there are just images—colors and sounds—being projected onto a screen that is flat and two-dimensional. Those flashes of color and sound form familiar images, so we see them as *a person* or *people, a house, a building,* and so on. As the images are repeated, we recognize the same ones again and again. Stringing these images together creates a story line with characters who become believable to us. In this way the mind takes form and color and turns it into something that seems real, alive, dynamic, and highly believable. And yet it doesn't really exist anywhere. It disappears once we turn the screen off.

It's still OK to enjoy the movie. *Just know that it is a movie*—a series of images flashing on a screen, telling a story played out by performers in costumes on a movie set, recorded in some other time and place. We can delight in the story even as we see through it. In fact, you might notice whether understanding that the movie isn't real somehow causes you to relax. It's funny, but when we see through the story, we often find new levels of meaning in it.

The movie provides an analogy for our day-to-day life experience. Mindfulness enables us to see through the illusion of our lives. Have you ever had the experience of creating a lot of personal drama and then later realizing things didn't happen the way you thought they did? A friend tells this story about watching the mind-made movie of her life: *While eating lunch one day, I was watching a father interacting with his little girl, and it led me into a classic "poor little me" pity party about how my father was NEVER around and NEVER did stuff like this with me. Later that day, an image flooded into my mind of my dad picking me up to go take guitar lessons together when I was a young teen. Poof! That was the end of that particular story. It was proven false, no longer relevant, and instead of being painful it became a source of sheepish amusement.*

It is very tempting to believe everything our mind tells us and be consumed by each and every experience of our lives. But this can lead to a lot of strong emotional swings—feeling happy, angry, sad, frustrated, jealous, afraid, happy again . . . which is pretty exhausting. With mindfulness we are *aware* of these emotions, we witness them, we know them, and we hold a little space for not fully believing them. The power of mindfulness allowed my friend to see through the story her mind was telling her. The result was less pain and suffering for her.

Renowned teacher Byron Katie suggests that with regard to our thoughts, we ask ourselves, *Is it true?* Once you answer this, follow it up with the question, *Can you absolutely know it's true?*

In a similar vein, Mingyur Rinpoche, author of *The Joy of Living*, likes to say, "Experience your sadness without really believing it." Sadness is real. And it is important to experience our emotions. At the same time, when we are mindful of our sadness (or anger, or fear, or worry . . .), we may begin to realize that frequently we are telling ourselves a story that evokes or perpetuates the emotion. As we listen to and understand this story mindfully, it may begin to unravel for us. And then, one day, perhaps the sadness is just an emotion we feel, and we don't have to believe it quite so much. It's just a possibility. We'll explore physical pain and emotions more closely in subsequent chapters in this section.

Continuity of Awareness

Beginner's mind gives us a taste of mindfulness. However, a bit of training is needed to experience mindful awareness more frequently and consistently. This can be developed through setting aside a little time each day for a formal meditation practice—time to simply pay attention. Taking time out of your day to sit, walk, or lie down quietly and just be mindful can be a big support in our work with jaw tension and cultivating awareness. As mindfulness becomes steadier, it supports calm and concentration. The mind becomes more organized, clear, and bright. It's a pleasant experience. On a practical level, regular mindfulness practice can help decrease anxiety, depression, and pain while increasing calm, joy, contentment, and ease of being. It also supports your capacity for mindful awareness throughout your day.

Cultivating mindfulness in your daily activities is *informal* practice. In addition to developing a regular meditation practice, awareness can be cultivated by simply paying attention to your breath and body at any time, anywhere, no matter what else you are doing. The combination of formal and informal mindfulness practice lends itself to a continuity of awareness. With concentration and mindfulness, we gain insight into our habits of mind and body—including jaw tension.

Mindfulness and Jaw Tension

Mindfulness is a powerful tool for health and wellness. As you cultivate awareness throughout the day, you might observe your jaw tightening in real time and consider, *What just happened?* Sometimes the cause of jaw tension is obvious—*Oh, I didn't like the way that person spoke to me. I felt criticized and tensed up in response.* At other times it may require more reflection to unravel the sequence of events that brought about the tight jaw—*Hmm . . . last week my coworker casually mentioned there were going to be layoffs. I realize now that was upsetting to me. What if I lose my job?* Either way, mindfulness helps you to notice when your jaw tightens and why it happened—leading you to understand cause and effect.

In addition to increasing your awareness of discomfort, mindfulness can help you observe what causes your jaw to *relax*. Our patterns of tension usually occur within a range or spectrum. There will be moments (or days) of tension and also times of relative ease. Learning what a relaxed jaw feels like is important. It gives us a target, something to shoot for. If you only know tension, it's hard to cultivate ease. However, once we know for sure what relaxation is, we can orient toward it with greater confidence. This will be especially helpful once you start to apply the techniques presented in this book. After using the guided meditations included in the audio downloads and doing the core actions and yoga poses, notice how they affect you. How does your jaw feel after these practices? Through the combination of mindfulness and yoga, you will learn about tension patterns throughout your body. Your personal body map (page 115) will help you to see how these patterns are related to jaw tension, laying a foundation for relief. (Review part one, Jaw Tension Explained, if you need a reminder of how the jaw is linked to the rest of the body.)

Mindfulness shows you the ways your actions impact you. When you see yourself repeating something again and again and realize it doesn't feel good, you can decide whether you want to continue with the same habit or perhaps make a change. If you have experienced addiction, you understand the power of this recognition. I have personal experience with this regarding my desire for sweets. A few years ago my doctor informed me my blood sugar level was high, in the range of prediabetes. It was important to change my habits quickly to avoid serious lifelong illness. I realized I had become a bit too addicted to buying cookies from the local coffee shop in the afternoon. In fact, my body even had an interesting way of telling me that it didn't want the sugar. My nose would get red and itchy. I had been trying to ignore this annoying consequence of my enjoyable habit.

Contemplating the doctor's advice, I realized I had a choice to make. I could carry on with this self-destructive behavior of eating sweets or I could listen to my body and use my red nose as a friend and wise teacher. I was the only one who could make a difference on this one—it was time for me to commit to myself. I decided to listen to my body. I realized my nose was keeping me honest. I could no longer hide even the smallest intake of sugar. With the incentive of keeping my nose and the rest of me happy and healthy, I began to investigate my sugar cravings. *What was I really hungry for?*

When the cravings came, they were really intense. And totally believable—*I must have chocolate now!* Every cell in my being wanted to get up and satisfy the craving. But I had learned there were some serious repercussions to acting out of this desire, beyond getting a red itchy Rudolf nose. Knowing the repercussions gave me a stronger incentive to resist. And even so, it was not easy to sit still and do nothing when the urge for sweets struck.

Drawing from my mindfulness practice, I began to turn toward the agitation. The first step was to become aware of my breath. Then I would soften my body and purposefully feel into what was going on. Just by creating space between thought and action, things became more workable. I felt myself calm down. And an amazing thing happened: The craving passed. I was still alive, most everything was still just the same—but I didn't have to eat that cookie, or chocolate, or cake. Even when people around me were eating all of these delicious things, somehow it was OK to say no, to practice restraint. Cultivating mindfulness of this particular habit helped me to stop harming myself, and there were other rewards as well. Remembering to breathe mindfully allowed me to stay present in my body. I realized I felt better eating protein, greens, or soup rather than running to satisfy the craving for a cookie.

The same principles can also be applied toward more dangerous forms of addiction. Mindfulness is a potent resource for changing destructive habits. As long as you remain unconscious, you have no choice. Once you are aware, the choice is yours. This is a profound step on the path toward health.

As Sharon Salzberg says, "Mindfulness isn't difficult. We just need to remember to do it." Mindfulness is available in every moment, all the time. We simply have to remember to pay attention. With clear intention and consistent effort, you can do this. As your capacity to pay attention increases, the ability to change your response to an experience or habit immediately, in any given moment, becomes readily available. It doesn't have to take a lot of time. Here's an example: The other evening I was completing an online assignment for a course I am taking. The homework involves many short videos, with exercises to be checked off electronically upon completion. I had done several in a row, including watching three or four videos. I thought to myself, *Well, I can do another, why not get more done? I'm on a roll.* In the very next moment I felt my right hip tighten up, pulling at my lower back. The feeling was distinct and sudden. I was tempted to ignore it and keep going. But that sort of pain was familiar and had more than once led to my lower back going into spasm. I began to question what was happening, pausing to notice my breath and take stock internally. Looking a little closer I realized I was pushing myself. It was getting late, I was tired, and it was enough for today. My body-mind complex was responding viscerally and clearly: *Don't push me! I'm ready to rest now.* I decided to listen to the inner cue. I turned off my computer and called it a night.

Mindfulness is similar to biofeedback, helping you become aware of what's happening so you can make conscious choices and cultivate greater ease whenever possible. It's unlikely you will be able to eliminate stress entirely, since it is a natural part of life. But you can develop a different relationship to it. Through directly experiencing your response to stress, making wise choices, and applying practices to support yourself as needed, you become resilient. Your range of ease and ability to recover from dis-ease expand.

You may recall the term *ehipassiko*, meaning "come and see for yourself," from the introduction. Cultivating mindfulness allows you to trust your experience and trust yourself. You are able to stand in your choices without doubt or uncertainty, because you know what you know. The principle of ehipassiko—trusting your own deepest experience—is applicable to healing jaw tension. With mindful awareness, you can unlearn the habit of clenching by directly seeing its causes and results and making wise choices in response.

To support you in developing a habit of mindfulness, all of the guided meditations are recorded and available for free audio download at www .catorshachoy.com. Each practice is also presented in greater detail in the chapters that follow. I encourage you to read about the meditations before you listen to the recordings, both for context and to know what your options are. Here is an overview of the mindfulness practices we'll be doing in the next few chapters.

Mirror Exercise

The first mindfulness practice is intended to increase awareness of your mouth and jaw. You will need a mirror to carefully observe the patterns of movement that happen when you open and close your mouth. It's important not to get caught up in judging your reflection (*Wow, who knew my lips looked like THAT?*) or trying to correct or perfect what you see. Here's an idea—try looking at your mouth as though it's not yours. Pretend it's someone else's face. Look on it as an experiment. The instructions are on page 207.

Oral Cavity Meditation

What goes on inside your mouth? Have you ever really paid attention to this? What does your tongue do? What about your teeth? Have you noticed what it's like to eat and chew food from inside your mouth? Mindfulness of the oral cavity is a powerful tool in our work with jaw tension. Three to five times a day, take a few minutes to be mindful of your oral cavity. For example, when you first wake up in the morning, at lunchtime, and before you go to bed at night . . . plus two other times. Doing this regularly will help you develop awareness of your habits of jaw tension. You will begin to notice when your jaw feels more relaxed and when it is tight or uncomfortable. As you become more familiar with your experience, you can start to ask yourself questions: *This morning my jaw felt great, at lunch it felt a little off, and now (at night) I have a headache. Hmm . . . What happened today at work?* With careful examination we begin to see cause and effect: *Oh wait, today the report I submitted was returned with lots of negative comments and a stern request for a rewrite. I'm realizing now I felt criticized and blamed and clenched my jaw to try and get through the day without feeling my feelings or showing that I cared.* This can lead to unraveling our habits of tension. Detailed instructions begin on page 210.

Three-Part Breathing

Three-Part Breathing is a potent technique for checking in with mind and body, as well as changing patterns related to jaw tension. In this practice we are purposefully changing the breath for a brief period of time rather than simply observing it. In this sense Three-Part Breathing differs from traditional mindfulness practice, which asks us to perceive experience without any alteration.

Three-Part Breathing gives us a way to undo the restricted breathing patterns often associated with clenching. It also helps you to notice *how* you are breathing and invites the experience of breathing freely—deep, open, long, soothing breaths. You can try this practice anytime, anywhere. Consider trying it whenever you feel yourself starting to clench: it may help you stop.

Once you are familiar and at ease with this practice, you can develop the Wave Breath, a natural next step. Instructions for Three-Part Breathing and the Wave Breath are on page 212.

Breath Awareness

The breath is always here and now. When we pay attention to our breathing, we know we are in the present. The breath is like an anchor or a rope to hang on to. It can be grounding, calming, and soothing to simply rest in breath awareness.

To demonstrate this, let's take one minute to be mindful of breathing. At the end of this paragraph, close your eyes, place your hands in your lap, and take three breaths. Notice the quality of each of these breaths. For example, is it deep or shallow? Smooth or rough? Is it easy to breathe, or is there some effort involved in pulling in the air right now? Try not to judge your breathing; simply notice it. From the perspective of mindfulness it doesn't matter how you breathe, but it is important you are aware. You might choose one word to describe each in-breath and each out-breath. For example, "short, long, smooth, rough, easy, difficult . . ." Are you ready to begin? Go!

What did you notice? (And again, remember you can't do this wrong.) Do you remember how you felt before the experiment? And how do you feel now? There's a good chance you feel a bit calmer, more at ease. Breath awareness is a powerful tool for calming the mind and creating ease in the body. Plus, you can do it in any posture, anytime, anywhere. Your breath is always there for you.

You can download this program's guided breath-awareness recording onto your phone or computer. Please use it regularly. Some of my students like to listen to it on their bus ride home from work. Written instructions (page 216) are also included to help you create your own recording or simply familiarize yourself with the practice. You really can do breath awareness wherever you are, for one minute, ten minutes, or a hundred minutes.

Here's another simple way to incorporate breath awareness into your life. When you first get into your car, before you turn on the ignition, take three mindful breaths. Do the same when you arrive at your destination: Before leaving your car, take three mindful breaths. Eventually you might start to take three mindful breaths before you change postures—moving from sitting to standing, from standing to walking, from lying down to standing. You will be surprised at how much you enjoy this once it becomes second nature for you.

Body Scan Meditation

The Body Scan is a form of meditation that takes your mind on a tour of your body from the inside out. This deeply relaxing practice can be used to unravel tension in your whole body and mind, as well as to focus on specific areas that are holding tension. I encourage you to use this practice for your personal benefit as often as you like. The guided audio and enclosed text are supports for your use. At some point you may find that your mind has learned how to do a body scan without guidance, and you might like to try it without the recording. The Body Scan practice has been used in medical settings for many years to help patients use the power of their minds for healing. It is a wonderful asset in the jaw tension program. Detailed instructions begin on page 219.

Loving-Kindness

Paying attention is an act of loving-kindness. It is important that we hold ourselves with caring attention, as opposed to with harsh or critical judgment. This might be called the double-edged sword of discipline. Discipline provides tremendous support in accomplishing tasks and living a life of meaning and value. Discipline can also be applied in a manner that is harmful or even abusive.

As you learn to pay attention, do so with love. Loving-kindness is a quality of friendship toward ourselves and others that is not possessive or controlling. Loving-kindness does not require you or anyone else to change in order for you to love or care for them. It is an open heart and a natural desire to help others, to share ourselves freely and to give without the need or desire for a reward or acknowledgment.

In the jaw tension program we cultivate loving-kindness alongside mindfulness to support overall health and well-being. Learning to love ourselves brings safety and ease. We naturally relax when we know we are loved. Listen to the guided meditation, and turn to page 200 for more info on this practice.

🌿14

Loving-Kindness Is Essential

Through loving kindness, everyone and everything
can flower again from within.
—SHARON SALZBERG

LOVING-KINDNESS is an attitude. It is a way of being in the world as well as with yourself. The Dalai Lama says, *Kindness is my religion.* This is a way of saying that we can choose to be kind. Loving-kindness is something we can cultivate and develop. And it is a very important ingredient in our work with jaw tension. What is held behind a clenched jaw? For many, there are unexpressed wounds here—feelings of fear or unworthiness, experiences we regret, a legacy of abuse and neglect, or harsh words of anger or blame that we were forced to receive or don't want to speak. The jaw is an incredibly powerful part of your body, as we learned in part one. Strong muscles can tighten and clench in response to emotions long contained, old memories never really forgotten. It may feel like there is no resolution. And yet this too can be worked out. Step by step, little by little, things change. We can learn to love ourselves. Offering loving-kindness to yourself is a way of creating safety. When we feel safe, we relax. When we relax, long-held tension patterns release. Freedom of body and mind results.

If you were alone on a deserted island, would you be good company for yourself? This question became meaningful for me when I went on a solo backpacking trip. After hiking to the campsite on the first day, I set up my tent, made dinner, and washed the dishes. Then I noticed the sun was beginning to set. Suddenly I became aware of my aloneness. *What would I do for the rest of the evening? It was only 7 p.m.!* To keep myself busy (and minimize my anxiety) I decided to take a photograph of the sunset at five-minute intervals. As I was doing this, I listened in on the dialogue happening within my own mind. There sure was a lot of critical commentary going on. My mind was filled with thoughts of what could go wrong, what I had done poorly, and what I should have done differently. Honestly, I wasn't being very nice to myself. Until that moment I had no idea how hard I could be to live with.

The practice of loving-kindness invites us to be our own best friend. Put another way, you are the only person you will spend your entire life with. Wouldn't it be more fun if you were good company? Ever since my backpacking experience, I've paid more attention to how I talk to myself, noticing the tenor of my inner dialogue. When I find that dialogue going downhill, becoming contentious or demanding, I make a point of resetting it. I do this by offering myself loving-kindness in that very moment. I purposely interrupt the negative communication with the loving practices that are included below. In the same way that I become uncomfortable with negative or degrading communication from someone outside of me, I notice and work to change these inner speech patterns in real time. I can still be hard on myself, but I seem to catch it more quickly. More and more, I see that how I talk to myself is reflected in how I talk to others. When I treat myself with kindness within my mind, I have more kindness to offer those around me.

As we grow in our capacity for self-love, it will naturally impact our relationships. Once we feel more at ease with loving ourselves, we spontaneously act kindly toward others. When we take this on as a practice, purposefully sending wishes for well-being to people we know, it contributes to our feeling of safety and interconnectedness. We begin to recognize that each one of us—every living being—is an important part of this world.

Sometimes we may find it incredibly difficult to love ourselves. In this case it may help to begin with the simple practice of forgiveness. Try saying to yourself, *I forgive you.* Anytime you notice a self-critical thought, *I forgive you.* Anytime you have thoughts of harming yourself, *I forgive you.* Don't give up. It's OK if you forget. When you remember, just start over. *I forgive you.* Notice how it feels in your body. *I forgive you.* Does your breath change when you read these words? Be mindful of the impact.

If someone has harmed you, you might try offering them forgiveness when you are ready. Do not force yourself to do what doesn't feel right. But there may come a day when you wake up and say, *I am ready. I want to leave the past in the past. I forgive you.* And then keep going until it sticks. As long as you are alive, the capacity to unlock your heart is available. Forgiveness can be the key that opens the door of your heart to bring relief from the burden of anger, resentment, grief, and despair. In many ways forgiveness is the precursor to, and lays a foundation for, loving-kindness. If you would like to explore the practice of forgiveness more deeply, a beautiful guided meditation from Stephen Levine is included on page 223. Stephen was a pioneer in this area. He and his wife, Ondrea, worked with people in prisons and confronting terminal illness. Their work continues to inspire.

With persistence we can overcome the painful experiences of our lives, breaking down barriers to love. With clear intention, our most challenging moments can offer us a vehicle for transformation and heart opening. For meditation teacher Tsultrim Allione, the journey of parenthood, with all of its inherent challenges, became a form of cultivating loving-kindness. She wrote about this in *Women of Wisdom*, published by Snow Lion in 2000:

> As I cooked in the cauldron of motherhood, the incredible love
> I felt for my children opened my heart and brought me a much
> greater understanding of universal love. It made me understand
> the suffering of the world much more deeply.

What experiences in your life have taught you about heart opening and universal love?

Eventually it makes perfect sense to extend loving-kindness to people we don't know and may never meet. Ultimately we can open ourselves to loving everyone equally, without reservation. We can even expand ourselves to send wishes for well-being to people we disagree with, we feel hostile toward, or who have caused us harm. Cultivating loving-kindness contributes to the possibility of a world free from violence, hatred, greed, and confusion.

Marshall Rosenberg, who developed a practice called Nonviolent Communication, takes an evolutionary perspective. He says violence is a learned behavior that developed over centuries, originating from a view of limited resources. At some point in the history of humanity, we began to feel more competitive, coupled with a sense that *there is not enough for everyone!* This is a message we have all received from society, through advertising, movies, television, and even our government. The bedrock of our economic structure is *haves and have-nots.* The myth that we are not all created equal is played out by worldwide economic and societal forces every day. Since we are a part of this global community, it is extremely difficult to extract ourselves from this view. In most cases it has also been reinforced on a familial level.

And yet it isn't true. There *is* enough for everyone. At this moment in time, there are enough resources on the planet for everyone to eat well, be clothed and sheltered, receive medical care, and feel they are a part of a caring community. What keeps us from creating a peaceful, egalitarian world? The anger, greed, and confusion of our mind. A simple lack of kindness toward those around us . . . which reflects the way we care for ourselves. Learning to love and care for ourselves *and* others is so important. Once we know how to be friendly toward ourselves, we have a better chance of bigheartedness toward others. Learning to love ourselves teaches us how to love others.

Loving-kindness cultivates a generous and compassionate connection between ourselves and others. This is different from a romantic or dependent love. It's more like what the ancient Greeks called *agape*, defined by St. Thomas Aquinas as "to will the good of another." In *The Four Loves*, author C. S. Lewis takes the meaning of agape further, describing it as "a selfless love that is passionately committed to the well-being of others." With this kind of love, we let go of trying to control others and instead accept people as they are, without a need for them to change or be different. Think how lovely it would be if we all felt a sense of kinship with everyone we met, all the time. Notice if your mind immediately rejects this as even possible. *Well, that's a nice way to think, but it's just not rooted in reality. That will never happen.* Don't give up before you have tried. We do not have to limit ourselves to what the world is today. We can imagine a new way of being. And we can take steps to create that reality—little by little, bit by bit, day by day. Look at what happens in nature: waves of water washing over a rock day after day, year after year, will wear down the rock in time. Profound change is possible.

In the guided meditation below, we will invite a loving attitude toward ourselves as well as people we consider to be friends, mentors, strangers, and eventually, those we have difficulty with. We can also share kindness and friendship with the nonhuman creatures we share this planet with.

The Practice of Loving-Kindness

Loving-kindness can be practiced anytime, anywhere. It really lends itself to being a highly portable practice and can be used in the moment for settling your mind. For example, let's say you're stuck in traffic. There's no way out of it, you just have to wait it out. Why not foster loving-kindness? Other great opportunities include waiting for an appointment, standing in line at the grocery store (I like to send loving-kindness to whoever comes into my line of sight. The person in front of me, the people operating the register and packing bags, the person in line behind me . . .). Yes, you can live this way, radiating love in all directions. It may be of particular benefit before a contentious meeting. Feeling agitated? Take a few minutes to run some loving-kindness phrases. It's especially lovely to practice as you are falling asleep at night—and it can improve your dreams and quality of sleep. And it also can be done as you are brushing your teeth, taking a shower, or making breakfast. These are all *informal practice opportunities*. They give us a chance to keep cultivating a positive state of mind no matter what we are doing.

Of course, it's helpful to cultivate a *formal practice* of loving-kindness as well. This is where we purposefully take some time every day to turn the mind toward specific qualities of love. It's best if you are not doing anything else during this time.

To begin, try spending ten minutes a day focused on sending loving-kindness to yourself. Do this for one to two months. As it becomes easier, you can start to share the quality of benevolent love with someone else. Below, you'll find categories of people—friends, mentors, acquaintances, etc.—to consider sending love to. Initially try spending at least one week focused on a particular category before moving on.

If you already practice meditation regularly, you can begin or end your meditation with loving-kindness. Cultivating love at the beginning of a meditation period can allow body and mind to soften, often supporting a calm and peaceful mind. If your mind is restless and you have difficulty focusing on the breath, try loving-kindness instead. Once you feel more settled, return to breath awareness.

There are different ways of nurturing loving-kindness. One method is to recite phrases in your mind. Another is through imagination or memories. Several options are offered below. I encourage you to try a variety of ways and see what works for you. Allow yourself to savor this practice. But if you can't—if you find you are struggling—you can switch to another category, return to breath awareness, or simply stop for now. Come back to it later on or tomorrow. Please be patient with yourself. Remember the cool water wearing down the hard rock over time.

Phrases for Well-Being

Let's begin by focusing on loving-kindness for yourself. Say to yourself silently, inwardly:

> May I be safe.
> May I be happy.
> May I be peaceful.

Repeat these phrases to yourself. Notice if your mind starts to speed up. Try to repeat the phrases slowly so that you absorb the meaning. This practice is not about rote repetition but rather about connecting to a particular experience. Consider how these phrases are landing in your being. If there are words that better express your sincere intentions, it's OK to change the phrases. For example,

> May I be healthy.
> May my material needs be met.
> May I be at ease in body and mind.

Find wording that you feel represents your real desire. You may even simplify it by choosing a single word that has meaning for you. For example,

> Safe.
> Happy.
> Peaceful.

One repeated wish may be enough. Three or four are plenty. More than that can be difficult to keep track of. If at any point it becomes difficult to remember the phrases, don't worry. You can always begin again or simply return to breath awareness. It's important not to struggle with this practice. Again, if you find yourself drifting off, take a break. Perhaps that is enough for today. Come back to it another time.

As a support for this practice, you might like to write your phrases or words on a piece of paper to keep on your bedside table, desk, or someplace you will see regularly. Alternatively, you could create an appointment reminder for your electronic calendar, causing your loving-kindness phrases to pop up during your day.

Well-Being for a Friend or Mentor

Think of somebody who it is easy for you to love and feel good about. This may be a friend or perhaps a mentor, teacher, or parent. Try to find someone with whom the relationship is not conflicted—a person you feel comfortable with and admire or appreciate. Perhaps they have helped you in some way.

It may be tempting to choose a romantic partner. You could experiment with this and also with someone where the love is more platonic. Notice the difference in the quality of your mind in each case. Do your thoughts become possessive? Is there a sense of love being limited in some way?

You could also use a pet. Our pets love us with such openness, they can be a wonderful model for what it means to love another being. The devotion of a dog, cat, or other pet can teach us a lot about love. The relationship may be simpler, less complicated; it's just about loving connection.

When cultivating loving-kindness for a mentor or friend or pet, it can be easier to see that love and happiness are infectious. This is one of the benefits of cultivating loving-kindness for the friend or mentor. Just bringing them to mind we feel our own happiness increase. We can start to see the mind as a love machine, generating greater and greater love for ourselves and others. As this love grows and grows, you may choose to simply use your imagination to start the love machine.

Notice how you start to feel as you envision boundless love spreading ever more widely. What changes happen in your body and mind? For example, is your body softening? As happiness and contentment arise, let your mind rest in this state.

If you have difficulty connecting to this visualization, you might prefer to return to the phrases we used in the previous example. Bringing your mentor/friend/pet to mind, say to them silently, inwardly,

> May you be safe.
> May you be happy.
> May you be peaceful.

You can choose any of the wishes from the previous section or make up your own. Continue this practice for several minutes, repeating these phrases to yourself, holding the image of your friend in your mind. If at any point it becomes challenging to think of your friend, this is all right. You can always return to sending the wishes to yourself or simply go back to breath awareness.

Loving a Neutral Person— Deep Down We Are All the Same

Next we will focus on offering loving-kindness to someone we don't know well and don't have strong feelings for. You might ask, *Why bother?* Cultivating love and compassion for a neutral person is an opportunity to fall in love with everyone. Instead of simply sticking with the people you care most about, you can embrace everyone equally—Regardless of how close your personal relationship is, regardless of their skin color or socioeconomic class, regardless of where they live or how they make their living. What if you truly loved everyone you met, all the time? How would it be to live a life of limitless good will and connection? Why not give it a try?

For this exercise, bring to mind someone who you run into periodically but don't really know. Maybe you know their name, maybe not. Perhaps you buy your coffee from them in the morning. Or they deliver your mail. Or they live nearby but you have never spent time together. Choose a specific person for this exercise so that you can clearly bring their image to mind.

This person is neither your friend nor your enemy. Bring their image to mind, offering them loving-kindness. You can do try doing this through imagery. Envision them as happy and contented, at ease in their life. Or you can simply share the feeling of boundless love, as in the previous exercise. Or you can return to phrases, saying to them—internally—*May you be safe. May you be happy. May you be peaceful.*

Loving-Kindness for Difficult People

Now we will direct loving-kindness toward someone who is difficult for you to love. This may be somebody in your life you struggle with, that person you "love to hate." You may feel this person has harmed you in some way, by being critical or perhaps even abusive to you. It could also be a distant figure, someone you don't know personally, like a politician or a cultural figure who represents brutality or cruelty.

Our natural instincts might be to reject this person, to consider them unworthy of love. However, I wonder if you would be willing to investigate this line of thinking. From the view of interconnectedness, we might recognize that everyone, even those who have done terrible things, has the same longing to feel safe, protected, happy, healthy, and peaceful.

Once you have chosen your difficult person, bring their image to mind and say to them, *May you be safe, may you be happy, may you be peaceful.* If you begin to feel resistance, you can return to sending these wishes to yourself or a friend—someone who it is easy for you to love.

Loving Everyone Everywhere: A Heart as Wide as the World

Finally, let's send wishes of well-being to all beings everywhere.

> May all beings be safe.
> May all beings be happy.
> May all beings be peaceful.

Let's begin with your innermost circle of friends, family, or both. Let your heart hold everyone in this circle. Send wishes of well-being to each of them.

> May you be safe.
> May you be happy.
> May you be peaceful.

Now let this feeling of loving-kindness spread beyond this circle, moving out through the walls of this building, out onto the street, touching everyone it meets with a feeling of well-being.

> May all beings everywhere be safe.
> May all beings everywhere be happy.
> May all beings everywhere be peaceful.

Keep letting your heart expand to encompass an ever-widening circle, spreading out across the city streets and buildings to touch everyone in the whole city.

> May all beings be safe.
> May all beings be happy.
> May all beings be peaceful.

Now let your heart expand beyond this city and across this country. Let your wishes of well-being extend across the ocean to other countries.

> May all beings everywhere be safe.
> May all beings everywhere be happy.
> May all beings everywhere be peaceful.

Let these blessings wrap around the whole planet. Let your heart open wide in all directions—above and below; north, south, east, and west; and all around. Let no living creature go untouched.

Exercises and Guided Meditations

1. Mirror Exercise

In this exercise you will learn about your personal patterns of jaw tension. No one has a perfectly balanced jaw. For an example of this, take a close look at the illustration of Lion Face Pose (figure 10.2). This illustration was drawn from a photo of my face. Can you see the imbalances in the mouth and tongue? Everyone has differences in tension between the right and left temporomandibular joints (TMJs). After a few weeks of doing the Mirror Exercise regularly, you will have a stronger sense of what is a "tight jaw" for you and what is a "relaxed jaw." While this may sound simple, in fact everyone has a range, and it is helpful to get to know your personal habits and tendencies within this range. Once you know the characteristics of *your* tight jaw and relaxed jaw, you can begin to observe what causes each of these. This may include factors in your external life—for example, what is happening at work, in your primary relationships, and in the world. What is your current stress level? Are you having any fun these days? It can also include body alignment and postural issues. How much time did you spend sitting at your desk last week? How much exercise did you get?

The most important aspect of this exercise is to remember that *everyone* has some degree of imbalance in the jaw, in the same way that no one has a perfectly balanced body. Don't beat yourself up for your imperfections. Accept them. Embrace them. Instead of trying to make them go away, recognize your imperfections as part of your unique beauty. Learn to work skillfully and wisely with who you are and what you've got. In Buddhism this is known as "the perfect imperfect." Or, in the words of Suzuki Roshi, *You are perfect just the way you are. And you could use some improvement.*

As you complete the Mirror Exercise, make note of what you see in your moon journal and on your body map. We will continue updating these through several more exercises until the pattern of tension you experience is fully mapped. This will lay a foundation for recognizing—and releasing—your tension pattern. Repeat this exercise weekly for a period of time to update your findings.

Stand in front of a mirror hanging on the wall. Imagine a vertical line down the middle of your face. This line passes between your eyes, down the length of your nose, and through the center of your lips and chin. Now open your mouth slowly. Pay close attention to two areas: the midline of your lips and the corners of your mouth. Notice these areas relative to the imaginary line you have drawn.

MIDLINE OF LIPS

As you open your mouth, notice when one of your lips deviates from the midline. Is it the upper or lower lip? One of your lips will pull to the right or left. Perhaps both lips pull slightly. Which one pulls first and in which direction? Does your other lip pull in the same direction?

As you close your mouth, continue to observe the midline of your lips. Does it return to center? Which has a stronger pull, your upper or lower lip? Open and close slowly several times until you feel confident about what you observe. Mark it on your body map.

CORNERS OF MOUTH

Now observe the corners of your mouth. This is the place where your upper and lower lips meet. Opening your mouth, notice which side opens wider. The shape will be slightly different on the right and left. A rounder shape is more open. A narrow shape is, well, less open. Open and close your mouth slowly several times until you feel confident about what you observe. Mark it on your body map.

Look at your notes. Does the lip midline pull toward the side that opens wider or toward the narrow side? Repeat this exercise, letting your gaze move between the lip midline and the corners of your mouth. Observe your patterns closely and make notes.

■ OPEN QUICKLY

Now open and close your mouth quickly while observing both lip midline and corners of your mouth. Does your pattern change with the quick movement? Is it a simple right-left or left-right pull, or is there a zigzag in there, with your mouth pulling right-left-right or vice versa in the progression of opening or closing?

■ JUST OBSERVE, DON'T CORRECT

The movement of your mouth is caused by an imbalance in your TMJs. Through this mindful observation of your lips, you are learning about which side of your jaw is tighter and which is more open. It may be tempting to jump ahead and try to fix things. *DON'T.*

It's important to simply notice what your jaw does. Rushing to correct an imbalance can cause a new pattern of muscular tension (a compensatory pattern) on top of what is already a compensatory pattern. That is to say: trying to correct your pattern at this stage can be more destructive than helpful.

Observing your patterns without immediately correcting them can be helpful in a variety of ways. When we get to know our patterns intimately, several things are happening:

Self-Awareness: As your mind becomes more familiar with its own habits, things will start to change on their own. This is the power of mindfulness: the brain builds new neural pathways. Through simple self-awareness, you are already beginning to heal. "Trying" to heal on top of what is already happening is over-efforting.

Mindfulness offers us a different, wiser approach. As we become more aware, we learn to react less, which lends itself to relaxation. Relaxation is a decrease in tension, which allows muscular patterns or compensations to dissolve. Body and mind come into a new alignment with greater awareness, which is beneficial in so many ways.

Nonreactivity: When we learn to simply observe something without correcting it, we are loosening our habits of self-criticism, blame, doubt, and anxiety. Nonreactivity is a potent skill for healing. When we release our judgments and biases, we open up to the possibility of simply letting go. The impact of this starts with ourselves and goes way beyond. You might be surprised to find that people start to feel safer around you as you become steadier and less volatile.

Letting Go: As our capacity for self-awareness and nonreactivity develop, something very interesting happens. We don't have to *try* to let go. It just happens. This is the path of mindful awareness. The mind catches our deeply conditioned habits more quickly, we see them, understand what we are doing, and realize how our habitual reactions are destructive to ourselves and others. And then we simply stop. Once we know how much harm we are causing, the letting go is a natural result of a well-trained mind.

OPTIONAL EXERCISE: WORKING WITH A FRIEND

If you are having difficulty observing the imbalance in your mouth, you may want to try this exercise with a friend. Additionally, you may notice it is helpful both to observe another person and be observed. Sharing your findings with one another is an important part of this exercise.

Sit opposite a friend. Sit close enough to see the movement of their mouth clearly. Take turns observing the movement of each other's mouth as described above. Then update your body map and moon journal.

2. ORAL CAVITY GUIDED MEDITATION

Oral Cavity Meditation can be done anytime, anywhere. The meditation can be done fairly quickly, in five minutes or less. Or it can be done slowly, over thirty minutes or more. My teacher Ruth Denison was famous for her guided meditations of the oral cavity. Sometimes they were so absorbing they could last for over an hour.

I encourage you to practice this meditation three to five times a day—for example, morning, noon, night, and two other times—for several months as an aid to unraveling your jaw tension. With regular practice you will gain awareness of your habits. Once you more easily recognize the difference between a tight jaw and a relaxed one, you can begin to notice what causes each of these. This is a key step in reducing jaw tension and the resulting discomfort. When we know what causes tension, we can learn to stop creating it.

As you tour your oral cavity, you will investigate the quality of the tissues within your mouth—do they feel hard or soft? Tight or loose? Heavy or light? Dull or alert? This is very different from thinking in terms of what is right and wrong. Right/wrong, good/bad thinking tends to lead to self-criticism and judgment, which are usually more harmful than helpful. If you notice your mind going in this direction, stop, breathe, and forgive yourself. This may sound simplistic, but it is important and entirely possible. Take a break, breathe . . . and experience any emotions that are present with mindful awareness. Forgiveness is fundamental to your health and well-being.

Sit in a comfortable posture. Begin to notice that you are breathing. Feel the way your belly stretches as you breathe in and releases as you breathe out. Let your mind rest here, following the movement of your belly for several breaths. Once you feel settled, bring your attention to your oral cavity.

Begin to study what is happening inside your mouth. Are your upper and lower teeth touching? If this is the case, then release your lower jaw down and away. *The upper and lower teeth should never touch unless you are actively chewing food.* Allowing your mouth to open may help to create some space between the upper and lower teeth. This is a simple change you can make anytime you notice yourself clenching.

Now let's investigate your tongue. Notice what your tongue is doing right now. For example, is it resting on the lower palate, soft and expanded? Is it touching the roof of your mouth? Is it pressing against the teeth at the front of your mouth? Or is it hovering somewhere in between all of these, tense and alert?

The tongue is the guardian of the mouth. Its job is to check out any object that enters the oral cavity and decide whether it should be there or not. For example, if you bite down on something hard, the tongue will find the object and push it to the front of your mouth, allowing you to spit it out.

The next time you are eating, notice how the tongue moves the food around within your mouth to ensure it is evenly masticated. This is a very important task that we often take for granted. It is actually the first stage of digestion.

The tongue is a strong and powerful muscle. It is instrumental in drinking, eating, nursing, suckling, kissing, and talking. If your tongue does not function properly, this can be a factor in your survival.

As with any good guard, the tongue will tend to have some tension. Notice the tonal quality of your tongue right now. Is it rigid, tight, or soft? Without any judgment, let your mind rest in the awareness of your tongue. Notice how your tongue changes moment by moment.

The tongue attaches at the base of the throat. Follow your tongue down your throat and perceive where it attaches. How does your throat feel right now? Is it soft, long, spacious? Or short, narrow, contracted? Notice the quality of the tissues. Is there ease or dis-ease? Often emotion can linger in the throat. Do you feel free to speak your truth in your life or are words held back, swallowed, or suppressed?

Follow your tongue back up to the oral cavity, and notice your teeth. How do your teeth feel? We can say that teeth are hard because they are enamel, but still there is a distinct quality of feeling to the teeth. How do they feel today: compacted, pressed against one another, tense, rigid? Or do they feel spacious, at ease? Run your tongue across your teeth to get a better sense of how they feel. What do you notice? Do the upper teeth feel different than the lower teeth? Is there an individual tooth that stands out and feels different from its neighbors?

Now let's examine your gums. Again, we can say that gum tissue is soft, but still there is a quality of feeling to the tissues. Run your tongue across your upper gums. Do they feel taut, rigid, or perhaps painful? Or are they cushiony, at ease? What about the lower gums? Are they similar or different? Perhaps the right side feels tight and the left side fluid?

And what about your lips? What is the quality of feeling in the tissues of your lips today? Do they feel stiff, narrow, tight? Or soft, supple? Is the quality of the tissues changing right now as you investigate?

Now let your mind once again fill the oral cavity. Experience the oral cavity as a whole. Does the inside of your mouth feel spacious, calm? Or tight, tense? What words come to mind to describe your experience?

When you are ready, allow your investigation to expand out to include your face. How do your cheeks feel? Tired, tight, rigid? Soft, open, expanded? What about your eyes? Your forehead?

Finally, open up to the sensation of your entire body. Feel your whole body sitting. Return to awareness of your breath, moving in and out of your body. Sense your belly stretching and releasing. When you are finished, make a few notes in your moon journal.

3. THREE-PART BREATHING AND WAVE BREATH

Three-Part Breathing practice is very calming. It can be done seated or lying down. It's especially nice to practice while lying in bed, first thing in the morning as you are just waking up and last thing at night before you fall asleep.

Since clenching can result in restricted breathing, this is a particularly beneficial practice for jaw tension.

Practiced regularly, Three-Part Breathing will inform you of your breathing patterns and help to bring balance over time. Once you notice your habits, you can begin to consider cause and effect. For example, *Hmm, I'm not breathing into my belly tonight. What happened today?* Through careful reflection, we begin to see how various interactions impact our breath and body. We learn what results in tension and what causes relaxation.

With this practice you will isolate your breath in three areas of your torso: your lower belly (below your navel), your upper belly/lower ribs (the area of your breathing diaphragm), and your upper chest (top ribs and collarbones). Each area serves different functions.

The lower belly is associated with digestion, grounding, standing on your own two feet, knowing and experiencing your emotions as they arise, sexuality, and sensuality. For women, we can include fertility and our monthly hormonal cycle. This includes menstruation, pregnancy, and menopause.

The first and second chakras are here (see figure 3.2). First chakra is located at your perineum. This is your root, your tether to planet earth. First chakra is associated with issues of survival: you are only concerned with yourself. For example, "Do I have enough (food, clothing, shelter, money)?" Second chakra is located at your navel and is associated with sensuality, sexuality, and relationships. Here we have awareness of two: self and other. When we feel threatened, we will often tighten the lower abdomen. For many, a soft open belly is a sign that we feel safe. Learning to breathe into your lower belly can facilitate deep relaxation and a greater feeling of ease.

The upper abdomen is associated with the third chakra: will, self-determination, community. Here we are conscious of three: How do we relate to a group? The physical structures in this area include your breathing diaphragm, floating ribs, thoracolumbar juncture, kidneys, adrenal glands, and psoas muscle origins. This area can easily become contracted under stress due to sympathetic nervous system activity—often called the fight-or-flight response. Tension here can become a self-perpetuating cycle of setting off our alarm bell system. Supporting this area to relax and expand can help to turn the alarm bells off.

The upper chest houses your heart and lungs. If this area is restricted, it will be difficult to breathe. When we do not breathe properly, many aspects of our health and well-being will be thrown off. In Chinese medicine, the lungs are viewed as the bellows that regulate the digestive fire. Reduced lung capacity can lead to poor digestion, circulation, nutrition absorption, and regulation of body temperature, among other things. Learning to consciously breathe into this area can even help to minimize asthma. (These are all good reasons to give Three-Part Breathing a try!)

The heart is the home of the fourth chakra. This is a gateway to the higher chakras. The heart is our refined feeling center, the place of alchemy where our coarse gut instincts are mulled through and distilled into the essence of connection between ourselves and our world. Opening your breath in your upper chest invites greater heart connection, improved health and well-being, and a refinement of your senses.

I recommend practicing Three-Part Breathing for several months as a part of your jaw tension program. Aim for practicing three to five times a day. In addition to practicing first thing in the morning and last thing at night, you can sit quietly during the day—in a chair, your car, anywhere—while focusing your attention on each of the three areas: lower belly, upper abdomen/lower ribs, and upper chest. At first we'll just do three breaths into each of these areas. Once you are more comfortable with the practice, feel free to stay as long as you want, but at *least* three breaths. For this practice you can breathe through either your mouth or your nose. *Initially I suggest starting to practice with your mouth open to be certain you are not clenching.*

◼ LOWER BELLY

Place your hands on your lower belly, under your navel. Your thumbs can meet at your navel, with your fingers spread out below. Pinkies can be close to or on your pubic bone. The base of each palm is close to your hip bone. Allow your arms to relax. If you are lying down, let your elbows rest onto the floor or bed. If they do not easily reach, then place a pillow, folded towel, or yoga blanket under them for support.

Begin by simply noticing the movement of the belly under your hands. After a few breaths, when you are feeling more relaxed, follow the out-breath all the way out, and with the next in-breath, intentionally try to isolate your breath in the lower belly. Refrain from breathing into the upper belly and upper chest. When you breathe in, allow your belly to stretch under your hands, pushing your hands up. When you breathe out, allow your belly to relax, causing your hands to drop.

Do this for three breaths. As you practice, pay attention to how your belly moves on the in-breath. It may expand forward, backward, and to the sides.

After three breaths, let go of any effort and return to normal breathing.

■ UPPER ABDOMEN/LOWER RIBS

Slide your hands up to find your bottom rib. Place your hands so that your palms are on your lower ribs and your fingers are on your upper belly. Allow your arms to be in a relaxed position. Attempt to isolate your breath in this area. Repeat as above, for three breaths. As you breathe in notice every small detail of the breath. For example, do the ribs move in all directions—forward, backward, and to the sides? Or are they restricted in some direction? Is there an individual rib that moves differently from the others? Or perhaps a rib that does not move? After three breaths, let go of any effort and return to normal breathing.

■ UPPER RIBS/COLLARBONES

Use your index fingers and thumbs to find your collarbones. With your index fingers touching your collarbones, let your hands spread across the upper ribs of your chest. Your thumbs will be near your armpits, middle fingers near your sternum. Allow your arms to relax. If you are lying down, support your arms as needed. Attempt to isolate your breath in this area as above for three breaths.

I'd like to offer you some imagery for breathing into this area. Imagine there is a balloon in your upper chest. This balloon is unusual. It is a magic balloon. When you breathe in, the balloon inflates. When you breathe out, the air leaves, but the balloon does not lose its shape. This is why it is a magic balloon. Also, this balloon has a limitless capacity to expand. Each time you breathe in, the balloon inflates a little more. When you breathe out, the air leaves, but the balloon does not collapse. Breathing in this way, your chest stays open, lifted, expanded even as the air leaves. When you breathe in, your chest opens just a little bit more.

After three breaths, let go of any effort and return to normal breathing.

Now rest and breathe in whatever way is comfortable for you. Take a few minutes to consider: Which area was easiest to breathe into today? Where was it the most difficult? How were you feeling when you began? How are you feeling now?

▤ THE WAVE BREATH

Once you are able to practice Three-Part Breathing with ease, you can attempt the Wave Breath. This is a natural next step. It can be done seated or lying down, after Three-Part Breathing or on its own.

Begin to notice how your breath travels through your body. The air moves in and out in the same way that the waves of the ocean move forward and back.

When you are ready, empty your breath all the way out. When you begin to breathe in again, let your breath fill your lower belly first, then your upper belly, your ribs, and all the way up to your collarbones.

Once you stop inhaling, hold your breath in for just a moment.

When you are ready to exhale, let your upper chest empty first—see if you can let the air leave, without your chest collapsing. Then empty your ribs, upper belly, and finally your lower belly. Hold your breath out for a moment.

When you are ready to breathe in again, let the wave of your breath fill your body, beginning with your lower belly, upper belly, ribs, chest, and collarbones. Hold your breath in for a moment.

When you are ready to breathe out, let the wave of your breath move out of your body from the collarbones (emptying without collapsing), then your chest, upper belly, and finally your lower belly. Hold your breath out for a moment.

Repeat one final cycle. Then return to normal breathing.

Here's an alternative metaphor for working with the Wave Breath. Imagine that when you breathe in, you are pouring water into a pitcher. The bottom of the pitcher fills first, then the middle, then the top. When you pour the water out of the pitcher, the top empties first, then the middle, then the bottom.

4. BREATH AWARENESS MEDITATION

Nothing can be delicious when you are holding your breath.
—Anne Lamott

Breath awareness is another meditation practice that can be done anytime, anywhere. For the most part, unless you have sleep apnea or you're intentionally holding your breath, you are always breathing. As a result, you can always develop awareness of your breath. Your breath is there for you, just waiting for you to attend to it. Breath awareness is a very useful habit to cultivate. You don't have to change anything in your daily activities—just intend to be conscious of breathing while you do whatever you are doing. Walking down the street, cleaning your home, watching TV, eating meals, reading the news, checking you phone, talking to a friend . . . you can still notice your breath. These are *informal practice* opportunities.

There are a lot of benefits to being aware of breathing as you go through your day. Attending to your breath will cultivate concentration. When the mind becomes concentrated, we feel grounded and peaceful. In a meeting, practicing breath awareness can help you to feel more focused. If you are in a conversation and things turn contentious or you're driving on the freeway and someone cuts you off, breath awareness can remind you to not react. Paying attention to your breathing also keeps you connected to your body— making you less likely to injure yourself or overdo it while you are moving your body and engaged in activities. You will be inclined to notice strain or tiredness more quickly and thus stop rather than push through and overexert yourself. Often, taking a few minutes break to sit or lie down and be aware of your breath can be enough to reset. You will actually have more energy and be calmer and more focused.

Cultivating breath awareness throughout your day supports continuity of mindfulness. With regard to jaw tension, this mindfulness will help you to notice when you start clenching your teeth or tightening your body and to let it go.

In addition to integrating breath awareness into daily activities, it's helpful to set aside time for *formal* practice. Around twenty minutes is ideal. In 1975 Dr. Herbert Benson published *The Relaxation Response,* with ample research demonstrating that it takes about twenty minutes of conscious relaxation for most people to settle their nervous system, switching from sympathetic *fight-or-flight* to parasympathetic *rest-and-digest.* If you can, establish a regular time of day and a specific space in your home for meditation. That will make it easier to develop a habit of practicing and help you reap the most benefit.

I encourage you to listen to the audio recording provided when you are first starting out. After a while the practice will become familiar, and you may want to experiment with sitting without the guidance. You can set a timer and use the instructions included here. If you just can't seem to find twenty min-utes, then try five or ten.

Put your body in a comfortable position that you can stay in for the duration of this meditation. You can stand, sit in a chair or on the floor, or lie down. Once you are settled, begin to notice the places where your body contacts the surface under you. If you're in a chair, feel your feet resting on the floor and your hips on the cushion. If you are lying down, feel the back of your body contacting the floor or bed beneath you. Let your face relax and your shoulders drop down a bit. As much as possible, allow your entire body to deeply rest and be supported by the chair, cushion, bed, or floor.

Now begin to notice that you are breathing. You don't have to breathe in any special way; simply observe that breathing is happening. You might sense the way your belly stretches as you breathe in and contracts as you breathe out. Or perhaps your attention settles on the expansion and release of your ribs with the in- and out-breath or the coolness of the air as it enters your mouth or nose.

When you notice you're breathing in, you might say to yourself silently, *In*. When you're breathing out, you might silently notice, *Out*.

In. Out. Just this.

Grow curious about the breath. How does it feel in each moment? Allow yourself to enjoy breathing. *In. Out. In. Out.*

What are the qualities of your breath? Does the breath feel shallow, or is it deep? Is the breath rapid? Slow? Is it smooth? Or are there catches? It doesn't really matter how the breath is. What's most important is simply that you notice it.

Let's try labeling the qualities of each breath as you sit and breathe. This is a way to be sure that you are really paying attention to each individual breath. For example, if the breath is short, you can say in your mind, *Short*. If it is long, you can say, *Long*. Just one word for each breath: *Smooth. Fast. Slow*.

Just sitting and breathing. *In. Out.*

Feel the belly expanding. And releasing. Feel the whole body breathing. *In. Out*. If you perceive tension building up, see if you can relax a little more and allow the chair to hold you. Let go of extra effort. Keep your upper and lower teeth separated inside your mouth. Just rest; sitting and breathing. *In. Out.*

When you find you are getting lost in thought, say to yourself, *Thinking,* and return to awareness of breathing. *In. Out.*

There is nothing wrong with thinking. We don't need to make it go away. However, it's useful to notice thinking. Try and have a bit more attention on your breath than on your thoughts. Let the thoughts fade into the background, allowing the breath to stay in the foreground.

Become aware once again that you are breathing. *In. Out.* Feel the gentle expansion and release of your belly or ribs or the coolness at your nostrils or mouth. Return to noticing the qualities of each individual breath. *Long. Short. Smooth. Rough.*

Take a moment to notice how you are feeling, even as you watch your breathing. Are there emotions present? Are you happy or sad? Do you feel calm or agitated? If this activates a lot of thinking, return to the breath. Your mental state may reveal itself through your breathing.

Just sitting, or lying down, or standing, and breathing. *In. Out.* Just this moment. Just this. Just this.

When you are ready to end, take a moment to consider how you feel now, compared to how you felt when you first began to practice today. What has changed? You may want to make a few notes in your moon journal. And then gently, slowly, get up and go about your day.

5. Body Scan Meditation

Body Scan (or body sweep) is a technique of running your mind's eye throughout your body with careful attention. This meditation cultivates mindfulness of the body and is particularly beneficial for relieving physical pain, which makes it useful in our work with jaw tension. The practice helps alleviate chronic tension, anxiety, and feeling ungrounded, replacing them with improved concentration and relaxation. The meditation lasts about forty-five minutes.

For this meditation, your body should be in a comfortable position. You can be sitting in a chair, on the floor, or lying down. Choose a posture you can hold for the entire time: it will be helpful to keep your body still for the duration. If you become uncomfortable, it's OK to reposition your body. Try to do so mindfully, maintaining awareness during your movements.

Begin to notice that you are breathing. You don't have to breathe in any special way. Simply notice that breathing is happening. Feel the breath as it moves through your body. Follow the length of the exhale and the pause that happens as the breath changes from out to in. Then follow the length of the inhale and the pause that follows as the breath changes from in to out. Notice the complete breath cycle—length of the exhale, pause, length of the inhale, pause. Find a place within your body where you can connect to the breath as it happens. This might be at your belly or the feeling of your ribs stretching and releasing as you breathe in and out. Notice the sensations associated with breathing.

Begin to notice the places where your body contacts the surface beneath you. Feel the pressure of your body's contact with the floor or the chair or your bed, wherever your body is touching a surface. Then begin to notice the sensation of your clothing or the air on your skin. Let your mind rest in this simple body awareness.

Now bring awareness to your feet. Feel the places where your feet contact the surface under you. Notice your toes, the soles of your feet, the tops of your feet, your heels. Bring awareness deeper inside your body. Sense the skin, and then the muscles under the skin, and then the bones. The bones are the densest part of the body. So we go to the bones, becoming aware of the skeleton.

Your feet contain many small bones. See if you can get a sense of them. Toe bones . . . foot bones . . . heel bones . . . ankles. . . . The ankle and the heel are composed of small bones stacked up to create the structure that supports the weight of the whole body. Perceive your body from within: feet . . . ankles . . . lower legs. . . . Get a sense of your entire leg: its full length, then the length of the thigh, the knee, the lower leg.

There are two bones that make up the lower leg. Can you feel this from the inside? Moving up from the lower leg, bring awareness into the knee. There is a floating bone in each knee. Try to sense it.

Next, feel the solid thighbone. This is the biggest bone in your body. Become aware of how the thighbone rests into the hip socket. Compare the right and left sides. Does one thigh or leg rest more heavily on the surface beneath you? Perhaps one thighbone is slightly rotated in the hip socket. Resist the temptation to correct it. Just notice what is so.

Keep an awareness of the breath even as your mind moves through your body, during the progression of this body scan. Observe your breathing as it happens, in and out.

Now become aware of the pelvis. How does the pelvis rest? Does one side rest more heavily than the other? Just notice the pressure of your hips contacting the surface under you. The pelvis lays the foundation for the torso, and provides stability between the upper body and the lower body.

Perceive all the bones of the body: Allow yourself to really get a sense of your skeleton. Notice your hip bones at the front of your body. Then follow the hip bones around to the back of the body, where the sacrum—the base of the spine—rests between the hip bones, the bones of the pelvis. Your spine extends upward from the sacrum, lifting up out of the pelvis. See if you can envision the lower vertebrae, just above the sacrum. They are about the size of your fist.

Allow awareness to move up the spine one vertebra at a time. Notice where the spine curves.

Now explore the base of the ribs at the back of your body. The lowest ribs don't wrap all the way around; these are the floating ribs. Above are the true ribs, attached to the vertebrae at the back of your body and wrapping around to your breastbone at the front. You might notice the ribs are not fused. This attachment to the vertebrae is actually a joint; there is gentle oscillation where the rib joins the back body. Perhaps you can perceive this even as your body is still—movement within the stillness.

Notice how the ribs hang, how they're suspended. You may feel that one or two are a little bit rotated or move differently from the ones around them. Or maybe they don't move at all. Perceive the individual differences of the ribs without any judgment. Notice how they change shape slightly with each breath, flexing and extending as you breathe in and out. Let your mind rest here, in the sensation of your ribs responding to the breath.

Notice the ribs wrapping around the body from the back to the sides and front of the body. Tracking the ribs all the way around your body from back to front provides a sense of the boundary between inside and outside, between your body and the outer world. Your skin is the boundary.

Bring awareness to the front of the body, where the breastbone connects to the top of the ribs. And then there are the collarbones. At the back of the body, you come to the shoulder blades. The collarbones, shoulder blades, and upper arm bones form the shoulder girdle. The pelvic girdle and the shoulder girdle are the widthwise containers for the body. See if you can sense this structure, feeling how things come together within the body.

Notice how the collarbones and shoulder blades are situated, relative to one another. Are the shoulder blades a little bit higher than the collarbones? Is one collarbone a little bit depressed, held down or back in some way? Or are the collarbones higher than the shoulder blades? Perceiving the shoulder blades, notice if one is a little bit rotated or held higher than the other. Without judging; simply noticing.

The shoulder girdle somewhat resembles the pelvis, with the thighbones resting into the hip sockets—but it is also very different. The shoulder socket is a shallow joint, with lighter bones and a much looser structure. Get a sense of how the upper arm bones rest relative to the shoulder blades and collarbones.

Then move awareness down the upper arm bones to the elbows and lower arm bones: two bones in the lower arms, similar to the lower legs. Notice the wrists, composed of many small bones, allowing for very refined movements. Wrists, hands, fingers. Perceive the skeleton directly.

Bring attention back to your breathing. Once again, follow the breath as it moves through your body. Feel your hands contacting whatever they contact. Just hold that simple awareness: *knowing touching, knowing contact*. Feel the weight of the hands resting.

And then travel back up the length of your arms, from the fingers through the hands, wrists, lower arms, elbows, upper arms, shoulders. Returning to the skeleton, feel the spine within your neck. Perceive how the vertebrae are much smaller here than the fist-sized vertebrae at the base of the spine. Here at the neck, they are about the size of the end of your thumb. Perhaps you can feel into the complex and delicate structure of vertebrae of your neck and how they interrelate with one another. The neck is a nuanced and sophisticated structure. Note the curve of the outer neck, of the neck's vertebrae. Bring awareness to the skull resting atop the spine. Sometimes the connection between neck and head feels very firm, as if the head were attached directly to the shoulders. What if you allow some space, some freedom between shoulders, neck, and head? Allow your head to rest lightly atop the spine. See if you can get a sense of that now.

Often we think of the skull as very solid, fused, hard, dense. However, the skull is actually very light. Some of the bones of the skull are so thin you can see through them. And there is movement to the skull, even when you are lying or sitting still. Movement within stillness, stillness within movement. You might begin to perceive that now. The skull elongates slightly and flattens slightly, several times each minute. This movement might be coordinated with your breath at this time.

Let the eyes soften and release back into the skull. Becoming receptive. No longer trying to see outwardly.

Let the throat and the tongue soften, becoming relaxed. No longer trying to express outwardly.

Let the ears soften. No longer trying to hear outwardly. You continue to hear because the ear functions; there is sound. And so you hear without trying to make it happen, in the same way that you continue to breathe without your own effort. Let the inner ear become round instead of oval, with a sense of depth in the inner ear.

Allow the skin of the face to soften, no longer needing to hold an expression. The face is the mask we present to the world. Allow the mask to dissolve, letting the muscles beneath the skin release any tension.

And then sweep awareness back down through the body, with a sense of clearing energy from head to toe, like a warm, soft rain pouring around you from the head, down through the spine, neck, shoulders. Arms, hands, fingers. And from the shoulders down through the torso, past the ribs, following the spine into the pelvis. Thighs, knees, lower legs, ankles, and feet.

Begin to imagine the air you breathe as clear white light. With each breath in, your body fills with healing light. If there is any place holding injury or illness in your body, send this light there. Let your entire body fill with light as you breathe in. And then sweep this light down and out.

Head, neck, shoulders. Arms, hands, fingers. From your shoulders, down through your ribs, your back, your spine, to the pelvis. Through the pelvis to the thighs. Knees, lower legs, ankles, feet.

Perceive the entire body as you rest here. Just sitting or lying down and breathing. Have a sense of the whole body, resting and breathing.

When you listen to the audio version of this body scan, the sound of chimes will end the meditation.

Forgiveness Is Possible

This essay originally appeared in the book *Guided Meditations, Explorations and Healings*, published in 1991. It is reprinted here with the generous permission of Ondrea Levine. Stephen and Ondrea participated in groundbreaking work supporting individuals confronting life-threatening and terminal illness, as well as working with incarcerated communities. They worked as a team, supporting and nourishing one another in this difficult arena. I am delighted to share this beautiful meditation with you.

Forgiveness Meditation by Stephen Levine

Begin to reflect for a moment on what the word *forgiveness* might
    mean.
What is forgiveness? What might it be to bring forgiveness into one's
    life, into one's mind? Begin by slowly bringing into your mind,
    into your heart, the image of someone for whom you have some
    resentment.
Gently allow a picture, a feeling, a sense of them to gather there.
Gently now invite them into your heart just for this moment.

Notice whatever fear or anger may arise to limit or deny their entrance and soften gently all about it.

No force.

Just an experiment in truth which invites this person in.

And silently in your heart say to this person, "I forgive you."

Open to a sense of their presence and say, "I forgive you for whatever pain you may have caused me in the past, intentionally or unintentionally, through your words, your thoughts, your actions. However you may have caused me pain in the past, I forgive you."

Feel for even a moment the spaciousness relating to that person with the possibility of forgiveness.

Let go of those walls, those curtains of resentment, so that your heart may be free.

So that your life may be lighter.

"I forgive you for whatever you may have done that caused me pain, intentionally or unintentionally, through your actions, through your words, even through your thoughts, through whatever you did.

Through whatever you didn't do.

However the pain came to me through you, I forgive you.

I forgive you."

It is so painful to put someone out of your heart.

Let go of that pain.

Let them be touched for this moment at least with the warmth of your forgiveness.

"I forgive you, I forgive you."

Allow that person to just be there in the stillness, in the warmth and patience of the heart.

Let them be forgiven.

Let the distance between you dissolve in mercy and compassion.

Let it be so.

Now, having finished so much business, dissolved in forgiveness, allow that being to go on their way.

Not pushing or pulling them from the heart, but simply letting them be on their own way, touched by a blessing and the possibility of your forgiveness.

And now gently, giving yourself whatever time is necessary, allow the other person to dissolve as you invite another in.

Now gently bring into your mind, into your heart, the image, the sense, of someone who has resentment for you.

Someone whose heart is closed to you.

Notice whatever limits their entrance and soften all about that hardness.

Let it float.

Mercifully invite them into your heart and say to them, "I ask your forgiveness."

"I ask your forgiveness."

"I ask to be let back into your heart. That you forgive me for whatever I may have done in the past that caused you pain, intentionally or unintentionally, through my words, my actions, even through my thoughts."

"However I may have hurt or injured you, whatever confusion, whatever fear of mind caused you pain, I ask your forgiveness."

And allow yourself to be touched by their forgiveness.

Allow yourself to be forgiven.

Allow yourself back into their heart.

Have mercy on you.

Have mercy on them.

Allow them to forgive you.

Feel their forgiveness touch you.

Receive it.

Draw it into your heart.

"I ask your forgiveness for however I may have caused you pain in the past.

Through my anger, through my lust, through my fear, my ignorance, my blindness, my doubt, my confusion.

However I may have caused you pain, I ask that you let me back into your heart.

I ask your forgiveness."

Let it be.

Allow yourself to be forgiven.

If the mind attempts to block forgiveness with merciless indictments, recriminations, judgments, just see the nature of the unkind mind.

See how merciless we are with ourselves.

And let this unkind mind be touched by the warmth and patience of
   forgiveness.
Let your heart touch this other heart so that it may receive forgiveness.
So that it may feel whole again.
Let it be.
And now gently bid that person adieu and with a blessing let them be
   on their way, having even for a millisecond shared the one heart
   beyond the confusion of seemingly separate minds.
And now gently turn to yourself in your own heart and say, "I forgive
   you" to you.
It is so painful to put ourselves out of our hearts.
Say, "I forgive you," to yourself.
Calling out to yourself in your heart, using your own first name, say "I
   forgive you," to you.
If the mind interposes with hard thoughts, such as that it is self-
   indulgent to forgive oneself, if it judges, if it touches you with anger
   and unkindness,
just feel that hardness and let it soften at the edge.
Let it be touched by forgiveness.
Allow yourself back into your heart.
Allow you to be forgiven by you.
Let the world back into your heart.
Allow yourself to be forgiven.
Let that forgiveness fill your whole body.
Feel the warmth and care that wishes your own well-being.
Seeing yourself as if you were your only child, let yourself be bathed by
   this mercy and kindness.
Let yourself be loved.
See your forgiveness forever awaiting your return to your heart.
How unkind we are to ourselves.
How little mercy.
Let it go.
Allow you to embrace yourself with forgiveness.
Know that in this moment you are wholly and completely forgiven.
Now it is up to you just to allow it in.
See yourself in the infinitely compassionate eyes of the Buddha, in the
   sacred heart of Jesus, in the warm embrace of the Goddess.

Let yourself be loved.

Let yourself be love.

And now begin to share this miracle of forgiveness, of mercy and awareness.

Let it extend out to all the people around you.

Let all be touched by the power of forgiveness.

All those beings who also have known such pain.

Who have so often put themselves and others out of their hearts.

Who have so often felt isolated, so lost.

Touch them with your forgiveness, with your mercy and loving-kindness, that they too may be healed just as you wish to be.

Feel the heart we all share filled with forgiveness so that we all might be whole.

Let the mercy keep radiating outward until it encompasses the whole planet.

The whole planet floating in your heart, in mercy, in loving-kindness, in care.

May all sentient beings be freed of their suffering, of their anger, of their confusion, of their fear, of their doubt.

May all beings know the joy of their true nature.

May all beings be free from suffering.

Whole world floating in the heart.

All beings freed of their suffering.

All beings' hearts open, minds clear.

All beings at peace.

May all beings at every level of reality, on every plane of existence, may they all be freed of their suffering.

May they all be at peace.

May we heal the world, touching it again and again with forgiveness.

May we heal our hearts and the hearts of those we love by merging in forgiveness,

by merging in peace.

❧ 16

Challenges We Meet along the Way

Working with Pain

We emerge into the light not by denying our pain,
but by walking through it.
—JOAN BORYSENKO

MANY PEOPLE afflicted with jaw tension endure chronic, significant pain that may extend far beyond their jaw, occasionally encompassing much of their body. Most often our instinct is to get away from this experience. Pain can cause us to tighten, withdraw, react. Chronic pain that just won't quit can lead to depression and really consume our life. What could possibly be good about pain?

In this chapter we will explore how to change our relationship to pain. Throughout the course of our lives, we all have pain at one point or another. It is a fundamental human experience and an important part of life, even if it is uncomfortable. Mindfulness can be a device for turning what we are trying to escape—in this case pain—into an ally.

I recall the meditation teacher Christopher Titmus asking, "Why don't we ever say, 'I'm cold, I think I'll take my sweater *off*?'" His point was not to invite voluntary suffering—though it may sound that way—but rather to encourage *investigation into what happens when we are discontented* and to experiment with what helps. How do we embrace the very experience we are trying to avoid? Life is not a bed of roses. We will all have unpleasant experiences; this is guaranteed. We cannot always escape from what we don't want. But when we work with our *relationship* to what we feel is unpleasant, pain becomes a powerful teacher. As we turn toward our discomfort, we may find a surprising result.

As I sit down, the first thing I notice is tension in my back wrapping around the right hip. This could be called pain. Instinctively, I press my lower back against the back of the seat and breathe. With the support of the chairback, I feel the muscles soften and relax, spreading out. Breathing again, things soften even more. And a third time . . . now my back is soft and supple. There is something so interesting about this experience. It pulls me in. My attention is total. Whatever was distracting me when I first sat down is now gone. My mind is happily resting in present-moment awareness. My humor improves. I feel at ease.

It takes a conscious choice to move closer to the experience of pain. When we make this choice, we are holding the question, *What is this thing I am calling pain?* With mindful awareness, you can break down pain into bite-size chunks.

Here is a mindful approach to try when you are in pain: First, investigate its characteristics. What are the sensations of pain? Is it hot or cold? Is it stabbing, piercing, a dull ache? Does it radiate or is it isolated? Perhaps images or colors appear with the pain. Reject nothing and embrace everything. All of your experience is valid.

Notice your body. Where is there tension? Are any muscles tight or gripping? Are you clenching your teeth or grimacing? Consider whether you might be able to relax a little.

Observe the quality of your breathing. Are the breaths short or long, rapid or slow, smooth or labored? Where is the air going—your belly, ribs, or chest? Try directing your breath into the place that is hurting. See if you can soften just a tiny bit, particularly as you breathe out.

Are there emotions associated with the pain? Or perhaps a particular thought or memory that repeats itself? Stay mindful of your experience. Explore the details of what you are feeling in each moment.

As you stay with the pain, it may happen that the sense of burden lifts. This is an opportunity to get interested in the *process* of what you are calling pain. Notice how the thing you are calling pain changes, moment by moment. Be curious about it. With body and breath as your anchor, you can notice fleeting sensations, emotions, colors, images, memories, and thoughts. Working with pain in this way, it may deconstruct and become something else. As we turn toward pain, it can happen that it actually becomes very compelling.

Strangely, when we are no longer resisting pain but rather examining it, it can cause the mind to unify around a single point very quickly. When the mind comes together in this way, ease and contentment result. How ironic that what we are trying to avoid—pain—can also be a source of relaxation, an invitation to drop deeper into being.

Once we experience this, we can use it as a reminder to soften to whatever we are resisting, whomever we do not trust, wherever we do not wish to go. It all becomes workable in some way. Even as we react, we can see another possibility . . . to collaborate with our discomfort. Through working with our mind's relationship to the situation, we transform the enemy into a friend. When we have no enemies, we feel safe. It becomes easy to relax anywhere.

Chronic Pain

If you live with chronic pain, embracing it might be more challenging. There is a deeply conditioned response, based in direct experience, to get away from that pain—more so than if you experience pain only occasionally. In this case, you may need a different approach. Let's start by focusing your mind in a way that feels easy. For example, place your attention somewhere in your body that is *not* in pain, like the back of your hand. Feel the sensations of the air touching your skin or the warmth of your hands resting on your legs.

If you cannot find a part of your body that's free from pain, then gaze upon a soothing image. A photograph of the beach, a forest, or the sky can work well. Any tranquil image is fine. If you have access to nature, this can also work: you can look at a tree, a field, or the sky. Soften your gaze. Allow your eyes to relax and rest back into your head—which means letting go of any tension and effort in trying to see something. Let your eyes, and your whole body, receive the image. Stay with the image until thoughts slow down and your mind feels more spacious.

Another approach is to listen to soothing music or recite a phrase that has meaning to you. (The Loving-Kindness practice on page 200 can be a nice alternative.) Notice your mind as you listen. As above, be attentive to changes in mental activity.

Once you feel calm and the mind is stable, then approach the pain. Start at the outer edge of sensation, where it's not so intense. Stay there as long as you feel at ease. If it becomes overwhelming or tension arises, then return to a place of ease through your image or sound meditation. Go back and forth between the edge of the pain and your stabilizing meditation in a way that allows you to stay mostly at ease. As you feel ready, experiment with gradually moving closer to the experience of pain. Don't push yourself. Let it come in time. Chronic pain may result from trauma but is actually a form of trauma in and of itself. As a result, we need to retrain the mind to not react to the pain. This happens through gentleness, kindness, and patience. It's easier to make friends when we feel at ease than when we are fighting. In time you can change your relationship to pain, inviting more ease.

The audio recordings included for Body Scan (page 219), Breath Awareness (page 216), and Loving-Kindness (page 200) can all support working with pain. While listening to these recordings, try applying the principles discussed in this chapter.

I sit with my grief. I mother it. I hold its small, hot hand. I don't say, shhh. I don't say, it is okay. I wait until it is done having feelings. Then we stand and we go wash the dishes.
—*Excerpt from* Taking Care *by Callista Buchen*

Difficult Emotions—Grief, Fear, Rage, Depression

The only way to deal with suffering is to be with it. Just allow it to be as it is, with a lot of softness. Be with your sadness and be with your joy
—RUTH DENISON

Life is full of strong emotions. On a daily basis, the pendulum swings from ease to distress to calm to agitation to grief to contentment to fear to peace. This is a part of the experience of being human and alive. In our work with jaw tension, it's important to notice the role emotions play in clenching and grinding. Mindfulness can help us learn how to accept difficult emotions and stay steady. In this section we will learn to apply the tools from the mindfulness practices offered earlier to working with difficult emotions.

At times emotions come on big and strong. They might seem like a tsunami, threatening to overwhelm and wipe us out. Then our fight-or-flight response kicks in; your instinct may well be to run and hide. But what if, instead, you stand strong? Imagine yourself like a pier extending from the beach into the ocean. The pier cannot run away. It remains firm through the worst of storms, letting the ocean wash over, around, and through it. The tide moves in and out. The pier remains intact. The poles holding up this pier are deeply rooted, sunk into the earth beneath the ocean floor. They are strong enough to withstand the surging tide.

Emotions pass. Even when they are powerful, we do not need to believe them fully. We might say things like *I am brokenhearted, I am terrified, I am furious* . . . but it is possible to *experience* emotions without *becoming* them. Experiencing emotions means feeling the sensations, knowing them intimately, becoming aware of the qualities associated with grief, fear, rage, or despair. You are not your emotions. You have emotions, but emotions do not define you. You are something much greater. Emotions come and go, like waves of the sea. They will pass. And you remain—steadier, calmer, and more confident for having known the intimate experience of the high seas of the emotional tide.

There is nothing wrong with anything. Have you ever said to yourself, *This is wrong! This is NOT how things should be! This is NOT my life, and NOT what I want!* And yet whatever is happening is just exactly what is happening. Our lives are not in our control. Emotions are a response to life experience and our relationship to what is happening. They can be uncomfortable. We may not *like* how emotions feel—the instability of uncertainty, the agitation of rage, the pain of grief, the numbness and burden of despair. However, the emotions in and of themselves don't need to be a problem. Mindfulness allows us to accept our life, moment by moment, just exactly as it is. Being receptive to your emotional experience without suppressing it or running away is what Jon Kabat-Zinn, the creator of Mindfulness-Based Stress Reduction (MBSR), calls *full catastrophe living*. If we return to the metaphor of the ocean, a boat on the surface goes up and down with the waves. But deep down at the ocean floor, things are calm. In the depths of your being, there is a steadiness even in the worst of storms. It is possible to hold the dramatic changes of your mind with wisdom, to welcome the broad spectrum of your experience. This clear seeing can allow for stability in the midst of the instability of life.

In the early days of the 2020 coronavirus pandemic, I was out for a walk in the neighborhood. I came upon a playground cordoned off with orange plastic fencing wrapped around the climbing structures. The swings had been purposefully tossed up over the top bar multiple times until they were wrapped tight and inaccessible without a ladder. To make sure no one pulled them down, they were wrapped in plastic. A sign hung on the orange fencing saying, "To prevent the spread of Covid-19, Baltimore City has closed all parks and recreation areas." Seeing the empty playground and reading the sign, my heart was pierced by our collective loss, as a community, a country, and for the whole world. Children and families don't play here anymore. I felt my stomach tighten, my knees grew weak, and I began to cry. This is grief taking over.

Stay with your body. Notice sensations. Can you describe grief? What happens in your body? How do you know it is grief? As you sit with the feeling, come up with a word or two that express your experience. This is a helpful tool to become *aware* of your experience rather than be consumed by it. With awareness the emotion becomes workable. Each emotion has a wise and connecting aspect. Grief is your heart opening. It is an expression of your caring and love.

> Reading the newspaper, I am impacted by stories of inequity and the resulting neglect of my fellow human beings, animals, and the planet. I feel heat and agitation building in my body. It's as though the ground has been cut out from under me, exposing molten lava. Tension increases, and it's difficult to sit still. Rage rises up in my mind and heart.

Notice your breathing. What is the breath of rage? Is it deep or shallow? Smooth or rough? Long or short? Breathe with awareness, just one breath. And then one more. And then one more. Gently, sit beside yourself. Hold your own hand. How does the breath change as you stay with it? Rage is a betrayal of trust. Within rage is the seed of forgiveness, the opportunity to let go of betrayal. If we allow ourselves to stay with our rage, it can be healed. Even as rage tells us it will last forever, rage can be resolved. Rather than trying to get away from it, see if you can turn toward it *with awareness*.

> Returning from a walk with a friend during the pandemic, I find myself sinking, drowning, as though I am tethered to a block of cement dragging me toward the ocean floor. I feel heavy, bur-

dened, and hopeless. Dullness and disconnection take over. This is really uncomfortable. Despairing thoughts fill my mind. I try hard to fight this experience. Then I give in, allowing it to pervade my senses. At the same time I am looking for a name, a word to describe what this is. After a minute or two I recognize this as depression.

Observe your thoughts. What is your mind saying? Can you be aware of your thoughts without believing them? One of the things your brain does is to generate thought. Thinking is a completely natural process. However, we do not have to *believe* everything we think. It is entirely possible to notice thinking and observe the nature of your thoughts without acting out of them. Create the intention to pause between thought and action to consider, *Is that really true?* The most painful aspect of depression may be the hopelessness that takes hold in the mind. By learning to observe this and recognize that it is simply a thought, we can begin to extract ourselves from the myth the mind has created. Breath and body awareness support this process. The loss of hope leaves space for renewal, for beginning again without controlling the outcome, without needing things to be a particular way. This is freedom.

At some point in 2020 I realized nearly all of my plans for the next six months or more had been canceled. It didn't make sense to create more plans with so much undetermined. In moments when I was alone, vulnerability regarding the tremendous uncertainty of this time revealed itself. My body feels shaky, alternating between tension and release, my mind feels fuzzy grasping at something, anything that might provide steadiness. And yet nothing does. I recognize fear is showing itself.

Please be tender with yourself. The truth is, life is uncertain. While we tend to live in a way that denies this reality, we never really know what will happen. The future is unknown. The events of 2020 only made more apparent a truth we like to hide from: *Life is unstable and unpredictable.* We cannot know the future. The past is no more. All we have is this present moment. Recognizing this reveals the instability of life in a new way. This can cause fear and anxiety. Interestingly, when fear shows up, it means we are not seeing things clearly. Fear is a form of confusion. Cultivating steadiness in the face of fear is an opportunity to let go of our small self. Holding yourself with loving-kindness can help you to feel connected and cared for.

Within the storms of life, steadiness can arise. Within the swirling chaos there is stillness. Dropping into the present moment, beauty is revealed in the mystery. Life does not need to be predictable. Steadying your mind and heart can help you to remain stable in the worst of storms. Everything is workable. *Just this moment. Just this moment. One breath at a time.* Try not to rush ahead or dwell on the past. *Just this.* Stay with what is here and now. Love yourself. Hold yourself with tenderness. You are not alone.

Mindfulness of breathing, body scan, loving-kindness, and yoga will support your capacity to be mindful of—and present with—difficult emotions. As your capacity grows, you may find you have the capacity to *respond* rather than *react*, during times of stress. This can lead to wise choices, resulting in less harm to you and those around you. This in turn leads to less stress and greater ease of being.

The Anxiety of Our Lives

Anxiety was born in the very same moment as humankind. And since we will never be able to master it, we will have to learn to live with it—just as we have learned to live with storms.
—Paulo Coelho

Anxiety is a uniquely human experience. No other species has developed their capacity for anxiety to the degree that we have. As a result, it is also a completely natural part of being human and alive. I have yet to meet a human who has not experienced anxiety. Have you?

Once we see that anxiety is unavoidable, the question becomes more about our relationship to it. Do we let anxiety define us? Or can we begin to look into the experience. What is it that happens when we are fearful? Tightness in the chest, sweaty palms, rapid breathing. The body might feel heavy or light, tingly or dull. What if we know our fear, rather than be consumed by it?

One time I was on a flight home to San Francisco from Boston. Just as they closed the boarding door, a summer lightning storm began. This meant we couldn't take off, nor could we safely deplane. We were prisoners on the plane until the storm stopped. The plane taxied around the airport until they put us in long-term parking behind some buildings somewhere. Three hours later, as we all milled around in the aisles, the announcement came we were cleared for takeoff. Within minutes I found myself squeezed into my window seat in a packed row of vacation travelers on a fully loaded plane with engines racing as we picked up speed down the runway.

And that's when it happened. My mind became obsessed with the exit door. Thoughts of how to get out of my seat and off this plane took over, racing right along with the roar of the engines as we hurtled toward takeoff. All I wanted was *OUT!* Claustrophobia arose, and a full-fledged panic attack came with it. The situation was decidedly uncomfortable.

What happened next was fascinating. I would have to say that mindful awareness kicked in. I watched my mind ask a series of questions. Question number one was:

What are you going to do?

This was a very good question. It was really tempting to react. An image of myself throwing a fit, screaming and yelling, climbing over my fellow passengers to access the aisle, working my way toward the exit door came to mind. It was immediately followed by an image of being tackled and restrained by the airline staff. *No, not that option. Next option?* This question gave me the opportunity to consider my actions and choose a less harmful approach to my dilemma. Even though some aspect of my mind was still in reaction, I didn't have to act out of that; it would only cause more confusion and pain for myself and others. Question number two was:

Can you breathe?

As it turned out, yes, I could. This presented a better option. I switched my focus from the precariously rambling thoughts produced by anxiety to body awareness. Once I did this, it was clear that the most difficult sensation was tightness in the chest. I began to gently breathe into that constriction. It softened slightly. The powerful practice of breath awareness helped me to relax a bit. The situation was becoming tolerable. In truth, most anything can be breathed through. When we stay with our experience, we find our wholeness, our refuge. The breath is a way to keep from abandoning ourselves in difficult times. It is nurturing and healing to simply breathe, one breath at a time. Taking deep, conscious breaths calmed me down. And then question number three arose:

What would help?

Now that there was a little space around the situation, I began to look for resources and support. *Connect to someone*, came the answer. I turned to the person sitting next to me and struck up a conversation. Turns out she was the nanny for the family in my row and in the row behind. They were returning from summer vacation on Nantucket Island. It felt good to hear someone else's story and think about something other than my own pain. I liked seeing how she worked to entertain the kids even though she was young and undoubtedly tired from getting up early for the flight and all of the other travel they had been through already. And she had also been on the plane just as long as I had and was working to create a good situation for those she was traveling with.

Eventually, as time passed, I was able to get up, move around the plane, and feel my body again. While the flight was initially uncomfortable, it became workable. I even enjoyed meeting new people. Further, it was inspiring to see that while I was panicked, the training in mindfulness I had cultivated over many years kicked in. Mindfulness allowed me to look closely at the situation, not be consumed by fear, consider options, and make wise choices. As I investigated the situation a bit more, I realized that as distressing as the anxiety was, *it was only a very small portion of my overall experience.* Fearfulness was narrow and tight, but mind was vast. What a relief to be able to orient in a new direction.

Working with Anxiety

Since anxiety is part of being human, it is worthwhile to learn to work with it, to turn your mindful awareness toward the experience of anxiety. I have found again and again that the three questions posed above help me reorient during anxiety. Anxiety wants action, so we are often prone to *reaction* in the heat of the moment. As a result, our actions may be poorly thought out or even cause harm to ourselves or those close to us. Even with panic it is possible to take a moment to consider what would be *wise action*. How can you best help yourself in this moment?

Turn toward your breath. Often anxiety is accompanied by a panic attack or the feeling that we cannot breathe. Slow down. Notice what is really true. What sensations are present? What qualities are apparent in the breath? Become deeply honest with yourself. What is your experience in each moment?

These two steps—pausing to review your options and mindful breathing—help to create a little space around the situation so you can return to yourself. The third—asking *what can help*—is really about loving-kindness. In the words of Marshall Rosenberg, founder of Nonviolent Communication, *What need is not being met?* As you stay with the anxiety and your moment-to-moment experience, it can be helpful to consider how you can help yourself. What would make a difference to you in this moment? Is there something you want to ask for or change? Pay close attention to the voices that speak within you. This is a way of befriending yourself. There may be a request from your heart.

Several practices and audio recordings included in this book can help with anxiety, whether it's situational or chronic. Three-Part Breathing (page 212) is helpful for cultivating calm. You can also practice it first thing in the morning before getting up and last thing at night before falling asleep, as well as other times during the day, to build resilience and step out of the habit of not breathing deeply that often accompanies daily stress. Body Scan (page 219) is deeply relaxing. Practiced regularly for a few months, it becomes more easily accessed and thus readily applied in daily life. Breath Awareness (page 216) helps us to connect to the body in any moment. In times of strong anxiety or panic, this is most helpful. Loving-Kindness (page 200) teaches us to be our own best friend, cultivating a sense of safety and belonging. Each of these practices support you to live in close connection to heart and mind. These steps can reduce anxiety and help you to live a more relaxed and peaceful life.

Mindfulness allows anxiety to be transformed into a powerful energy of fearlessness and connection—not through pushing through but rather by accepting and patiently, gently, getting to know it better. Audre Lorde, the apparently fearless African American civil rights activist and poet, put it this way in *The Transformation of Silence into Language and Action*:

> I began to recognize a source of power within myself that comes
> from the knowledge that while it is most desirable not to be afraid,
> learning to put fear into a perspective gave me great strength.

Appendix: Moon Journal Resources

A moon journal can be a wonderful support for healing from jaw tension. Use it to record your daily experience of your jaw and any other symptoms, as well as what practices you are applying. It's also helpful to include unusual events—for example, diet changes, travel, excessive work schedule, dramatic weather, and so on. For women, including your hormonal cycle will be helpful. Tuning in to the rhythm of the moon is beneficial for everyone, regardless of gender. After a few months of recording information in your journal, look back and see whether patterns emerge for you regarding the symptoms you experience. This often appears over a period of three to six months. Seeing these patterns can help to understand cause and effect, which can lay a foundation for unraveling destructive or painful habits. Keeping a moon journal can bring us closer to nature—and interbeing. The waxing and waning of La Luna reminds us of how connected we are to our environment and that we cannot fully separate ourselves from everyone and everything around us. Understanding this, we can cultivate a wise relationship toward body and mind. Below is a list of my favorite moon journals.

- If you are in a coastal area, a tide log combines the tides with moon phases: www.tidelog.com.
- This single-page lunar phase calendar for the entire year is a lovely poster, which can be used in combination with a conventional journal: www.equinoxastrology.com/moon.
- We Moon offers a delightful range of lunar calendars: https://wemoon.ws.
- The Old Farmer's Almanac carries month calendars and daily planners that display the phases of the moon: https://store.almanac.com /calendars.

- Etsy is home to a wide variety of independent artists creating lunar calendars: www.etsy.com.
- There are also many other apps and online resources for moon phase calendars and journals.

Notes

Chapter 1: Jaw Tension Defined

1. Neil S. Norton, *Netter's Head and Neck Anatomy for Dentistry* (London: Elsevier Health Sciences, 2016), 251; Lígia Figueiredo Valesan et al., "Prevalence of Temporomandibular Joint Disorders: A Systematic Review and Meta-Analysis," *Clinical Oral Investigation* 25, no. 2 (February 2021): 441–53.

2. Caroline Bueno et al., "Gender Differences in Temporomandibular Disorders in Adult Populational Studies: A Systemic Review and Meta-Analysis," *Journal of Oral Rehabilitation* 45, no. 9 (2018): 720–29.

3. Sumit Yadav et al., "Tempormandibular Joint Disorders in Older Adults," *Journal of American Geriatric Society* 66, no. 6 (2018): 1213–17.

4. Nikolaus Christidis et al., "Prevalence and Treatment Strategies Regarding Temporomandibular Disorders in Children and Adolescents: A Systemic Review," *Journal of Oral Rehabilitation* 46, no.3 (2019): 291–301.

5. Viola M. Frymann, "Relation of Disturbances of craniosacral Mechanism to Symptomology of the Newborn: Study of 1,250 Infants," *Journal of the American Osteopathic Association* 65 (1966): 1059–75; republished by American Academy of Osteopathy 1998.

Chapter 2: Anatomy of Your Jaw

1. Stephen Wroe et al., "The Craniomandibular Mechanics of Being Human," *Proceedings of the Royal Society B* 277, no. 1700 (December 7, 2010): 3579–86.

2. Yoshinobu Ide and K. Nakazawa, *Anatomical Atlas of the Temporomandibular Joint* (Batavia, IL: Quintessence Publishing, 1991).

3. Aelred C. Fonder, *Dental Distress Syndrome* (Chicago: Medical-Dental Arts, 1990): 12–13.

4. Hugh Milne, *The Heart of Listening*, vol. 2 (Berkeley, CA: North Atlantic Books, 1998), 23.

5. Christopher Ruff et al., "Who's afraid of the big bad Wolff?: 'Wolff's law' and bone functional adaptation," *American Journal of Physical Anthropology* 129, no. 4 (April 2006): 484–98.

6. James Pampush and David J. Daegling, "The Enduring Puzzle of the Human Chin," *Evolutionary Anthropology* 25, no. 1 (January 2016): 20–35.

7. Robert Seigel, Why Do Humans Have Chins? A Scientist Explains the 'Enduring Puzzle,' *All Things Considered, NPR,* January 29, 2016, https://www.npr.org/2016/01/29/464893281/why-do-humans-have-chins-a-scientist-explains-the-enduring-puzzle.

8. Sandra Kahn and Paul R. Ehrlich, *Jaws: The Story of a Hidden Epidemic* (Palo Alto, CA: Stanford University Press, 2018).

9. Weston A. Price, *Nutrition and Physical Degeneration* (Lemon Grove, CA: Price-Pottenger, 1939).

10. Milne, *The Heart of Listening*, vol. 2, 169.

11. James Nestor, *Breath* (New York: Riverhead Books, 2021).

12. Kahn and Ehrlich, *Jaws.*

13. Peter W. Alberti, "The Anatomy and Physiology of the Ear and Hearing" (paper), University of Singapore, Department of Ontolaryngology, https://www.who.int/occupational_health/publications/noise2.pdf).

14. Fonder, *Dental Distress Syndrome.*

15. Milne, *The Heart of Listening*, vol. 2, 121.

16. Frymann, "Relation of Disturbances."

17. Fonder, *Dental Distress Syndrome.*

18. Stephen Porges, "The Role of Social Engagement in Attachment and Bonding: A Phylogenetic Perspective," chapter 3 in *Attachment and Bonding: A New Synthesis*, ed. C. Sue Carter et al. (Cambridge, MA: MIT Press, 2005).

19. Ide and Nakazawa, *Anatomical Atlas*, 112.

20. Maulana Jalāl al-Dīn Rūmī, "The Breeze at Dawn," in *The Essential Rumi*, trans. Coleman Barks (New York: HarperCollins, 1996), 36. Reprinted with permission.

21. Franklyn Sills, *Craniosacral Biodynamics*, vol. 2 (Berkeley, CA: North Atlantic Books, 2004), chapter 15.

Chapter 3: The Inner Tide and Cranial Wave

1. Frymann, "A Study of the Rhythmic Motions of the Living Cranium," *Journal of the American Osteopathic Association* 70 (May 1971): 928–45. NB: Numerous studies have been conducted verifying cranial motility. See Richard A. Feely, ed., *Clinical Cranial Osteopathy* (Leawood, KS: Osteopathic Cranial Academy, 1988). This book collects and republishes earlier research. Additionally, the more recent publication by Michael Kern, *Wisdom in the Body* (Berkeley, CA: North Atlantic Books, 2001), offers detailed research information regarding cranial movement.

2. Sills, *Craniosacral Biodynamics*, vols. 1–2; Milne, *The Heart of Listening vol. 1–2*; Kern, *Wisdom in the Body.*

3. Note: The three references above also detail long tide.

4. Adah Strand Sutherland, *With Thinking Fingers* (Leawood, KS: Osteopathic Cranial Academy, 1962), chapter 3.

5. Sutherland, *With Thinking Fingers.*

6. Sutherland, *With Thinking Fingers.*

7. Sutherland, *With Thinking Fingers.*

8. Frymann, "A Study of the Rhythmic Motions of the Living Cranium."

9. Vasant Lad, *The Textbook of Ayurveda Fundamental Principles* (Albuquerque, NM: Ayur-

vedic Press, 2002). NB: Information on the vayus (*rlung* in Tibetan) appears in numerous books on Indian and Tibetan Ayurveda. Occasionally names of the individual vayus will differ. This is recognized as an inconsistency within Indian Ayurveda. The Tibetan system appears to be more consistent. Other publications to reference include: David Frawley, *Yoga and Ayurveda* (Detroit, MI: Lotus Press, 1999); Yeshe Donden, *Healing through Balance* (Ithaca, NY: Snow Lion Publications, 1986); Yeshe Donden and Jhampa Kelsang, *Healing from the Source* (Ithaca, NY: Snow Lion Publications, 2000).

Chapter 4: Dental Work and TMD

1. Bessel A. van der Kolk, *The Body Keeps the Score: Brain, Mind, and Body in the Healing of Trauma* (New York: Penguin, 2015).
2. Fonder, *The Dental Distress Syndrome*, 93.
3. Fonder, *The Dental Distress Syndrome*, 93.

Chapter 5: Your Ears and Your Jaw

1. Ide and Nakazawa, *Anatomical Atlas*, 15.
2. William G. Sutherland, *Contributions of Thought: The Collected Writings of William Garner Sutherland* (Portland, OR: Rudra Press, 1997), chapter 27.
3. James R. Hagerty, "Texas Roadhouse CEO Kent Taylor, a Business Maverick, Was Tormented by Tinnitus after Covid-19," *Wall Street Journal*, March 24, 2021.
4. Stephen W. Porges, *The Pocket Guide to the Polyvagal Theory* (New York: W. W. Norton, 2017).
5. Bryan Pietsch, "Kent Taylor, Texas Roadhouse Founder and C.E.O., Dies at 65," *New York Times*, March 21, 2021.
6. Darius Marder, dir. *The Sound of Metal* (Culver City, CA: Amazon Studios 2020).

Chapter 6: Headaches, Stress, Trauma, and TMD

1. Kelly McGonigal, *The Upside of Stress* (New York: Penguin Random House, 2016).
2. Porges, *The Pocket Guide to the Polyvagal Theory*.
3. Porges, "The Role of Social Engagement in Attachment and Bonding."
4. Freddy Drabble (host), "Polyvagal Theory Explained with Stephen Porges, PhD." episode 5, *Chasing Consciousness*, audio/video podcast, May 31, 2021, https://www.chasingconsciousness.net/episodes.
5. Karin Roelofs, "Freeze for Action: Neurobiological Mechanisms in Animal and Human Freezing," *Philosophical Transactions of the Royal Society B* 372, no. 1718 (April 2017).
6. Migraineresearchfoundation.org.
7. Sabrina Khan et al., "Meningeal Contribution to Migraine Pain: A Magnetic Resonance Angiography Study," *Brain* 142, no. 1 (Jan. 2019): 93–102.
8. Smriti Iyengar et al., "CGRP and the Trigeminal System in Migraine," *Headache* 59, no. 5 (May 2019): 659–81.
9. Bianca N. Mason et al., "Vascular Contributions to Migraine: Time to Revisit?" *Frontiers in Cellular Neuroscience* 12 (2018): 233.

10. Dale Purves et al., "The Blood Supply of the Brain and Spinal Cord," in *Neuroscience* 2nd ed. (Sunderland, MA: Sinauer Associates, 2001).

11. Erin P. Fillmore et al., "Anatomy of the Trigeminal Nerve," vol. 1, *History, Embryology, Anatomy, Imaging, and Diagnostics*, ed. R. Shane Tubbs et al. (London: Academic Press, 2015).

12. Matthew S. Robbins et al., "The Sphenopalatine Ganglion: Anatomy, Pathophysiology and Therapeutic Targeting in Headache," *Headache* 56, no. 2 (February 2016): 240–58.

13. William Garner Sutherland, *The Cranial Bowl* (Leawood, KS: The Osteopathic Cranial Academy, 1939), 115–16.

14. Jennifer L. Robinson et al., "Estrogen Signaling Impacts Temporomandibular Joint and Periodontal Disease Pathology," *Odontology* 108, no. 2 (April 2020): 153–65.

15. Sills, *Craniosacral Biodynamics*, vol.2, Intraosseous Occipital Distortions, 120–21, chapters 14, 15, 16.

Chapter 7: Hips, Feet, Hypermobility, and Your Jaw

1. Nestor, *Breath*.

2. Krzysztof A. Tomaszewski et al., "A Surgical Anatomy of the Sciatic Nerve: A Meta-Analysis," *Journal of Orthopaedic Research* 34, no. 10 (Oct. 2016): 1820–27.

3. Bruno Bordoni et al., "Tentorium Cerebelli: Muscles, Ligaments and Dura Mater, Part 1," *Cureus* 11, no. 9 (September, 2019): e5601

4. Note: The dural tube upper attachments are at foramen magnum, C2 and C3. Lower attachments are at the second sacral segment and end of the tailbone, called *filum terminalis*. There are minor attachments at the lumbar vertebrae. This is referenced in numerous anatomical textbooks, including Frank H. Netter, *Atlas of Human Anatomy* (London: Elsevier, 1997).

5. Sutherland, *Contributions of Thought*, chapters 17 and 27.

6. Sutherland, *Teaching in the Science of Osteopathy* (Portland, OR: Sutherland Cranial Teaching Foundation, 1990), chapter 4.

7. Sutherland, *The Cranial Bowl*, 45–46.

8. Harold Ives Magoun, *Osteopathy in the Cranial Field* (Kirksville, MO: Osteopathic Cranial Association, 1951), chapter 1.

9. Sills, *Craniosacral Biodynamics*, vol. 2, Formative Forces and Mid-lines.

10. Cindy C. Sangalang and Cindy Vang, "Intergenerational Trauma in the Refugee Families: A Systematic Review," *Journal of Immigrant and Minority Health* 19, no. 3 (June 2017): 745–54.

11. Tori DeAngelis, "The Legacy of Trauma—an Emerging Line of Research Is Exploring How Historical and Cultural Traumas Affect Survivors' Children for Generations to Come," *American Psychological Association* 50, no. 2 (Feb. 2019): 36.

Chapter 8: Conscious Healing Touch Facial Self-Massage for TMD

1. Tiffany Field, *Touch* (Cambridge, MA: MIT Press, 2003).

2. Crystal Cox, "People Are Experiencing Skin Hunger After Months Without Touching Anyone," June 9, 2020, Insider.com.

3. Maham Hasan, "What All That Touch Deprivation Is Doing to Us," *New York Times*, October 6, 2020.

4. Suzanne Degges-White, "Skin Hunger, Touch Starvation and Hug Deprivation," *Psychology Today*, November 20, 2020.

5. Kirsten Weir, "The Lasting Impact of Neglect," *American Psychological Association* 45, no. 6 (June 2014): 36.

6. Melissa Fay Greene, "30 Years Ago, Romania Deprived Thousands of Babies of Human Contact," *The Atlantic*, June 23, 2020.

7. Université Laval, "Preemies' Brains Reap Long-Term Benefits from Kangaroo Mother Care," *ScienceDaily*, September 19, 2012, www.sciencedaily.com/releases/2012/09/120919125600 .htm.

8. Francis McGlone et al., "Discriminative and Affective Touch: Sensing and Feeling," *Neuron* 82, no. 4 (May 2014): 737–55.

Chapter 9: Getting Started

1. National Center for Complimentary and Integrative Health, "Yoga: What You Need to Know," accessed September 19, 2021, https://www.nccih.nih.gov/health/yoga-what-you-need-to -know.

2. Note: The research demonstrating the efficacy of mindfulness for a wide range of health benefits is so vast, it's hard to find a single citation that adequately expresses this body of work. To date there are reportedly upwards of two thousand high-quality studies on the subject. Here are a few easily accessible resources that cite significant published research papers, including leading university research websites and a literature review:

   Center for Healthy Minds, University of Wisconsin Madison, accessed September 18, 2021, https://centerhealthyminds.org/science/research.

   Shian-Ling Keng et al., "Effects of Mindfulness on Psychological Health: A Review of Empirical Studies," *Clinical Psychology Review* 31, no. 6 (Aug. 2011): 1041–56.

   Jill Suttie, "Five Ways Mindfulness is Good for Your Health," Greater Good Science Center, October 24, 2018, https://greatergood.berkeley.edu/article/item/five_ways_mindfulness_ meditation_is_good_for_your_health.

   UCLA Mindful Awareness Research Center (MARC), accessed September 18, 2021, https://www.uclahealth.org/marc/research.

3. Per Trobisch et al, "Idiopathic Scoliosis," *Deutsches Ärzteblatt International* 107, no. 49 (December 2010): 875–83.

4. Linda J. Dimitroff, et al. "Changing Your Life Through Journaling—the Benefits of Journaling for Registered Nurses," *Journal of Nursing Education and Practice* 7, no. 2 (2017): 90–98; Maud Purcell, "The Health Benefits of Journaling," *PsychCentral*, May 17, 2016, https://psychcentral.com/lib/the-health-benefits-of-journaling#1.

Bibliography

Articles and Research Papers

Bordoni, Bruno, Marta Simonelli, and Maria Marcella Lagana. "Tentorium Cerebelli: Muscles, Ligaments, and Dura Mater, Part 1." *Cureus* 11, no. 9 (September 2019): e5601.

Bueno, Caroline H., Duziene D. Pereira, Marcos Pascoal Pattusi, Patricia Krieger Grossi, and Marcio L. Grossi. "Gender Differences in Temporomandibular Disorders in Adult Populational Studies: A Systematic Review and Meta-Analysis." *Journal of Oral Rehabilitation* 45, no. 9 (2018): 720–29.

Christidis, Nikolaos, Elisande Lindstrom Ndanshau, Amanda Sandberg, and Georgios Tsilingaridis. "Prevalence and Treatment Strategies Regarding Temporomandibular Disorders in Children and Adolescents: A Systemic Review." *Journal of Oral Rehabilitation* 46, no. 3 (2019): 291–301.

Cox, Crystal. "People Are Experiencing 'Skin Hunger' after Months without Touching Anyone." Insider.com, June 9, 2020.

DeAngelis, Tori. "The Legacy of Trauma—an Emerging Line of Research Is Exploring How Historical and Cultural Traumas Affect Survivors' Children for Generations to Come." *American Psychological Association* 50, no. 2 (February 2019): 36.

Degges-White, Suzanne. "Skin Hunger, Touch Starvation, and Hug Deprivation." *Psychology Today*, November 20, 2020.

Dimitroff, Lynda J., Linda Sliwoski, Sue O'Brien, and Lynn W. Nichols. "Changing Your Life through Journaling—the Benefits of Journaling for Registered Nurses." *Journal of Nursing Education and Practice* 7, no. 2 (2017): 90–98.

Fillmore, Erin P., and Mark F. Seifert. "Anatomy of the Trigeminal Nerve." In *Nerves and Nerve Injuries*, vol. 1, *History Embryology, Anatomy, Imaging, and Diagnostics*, edited by R. Shane Tubbs, Elias Rizk, Mohammadali M. Shoja, Marios Loukas, Nicholas Barbaro, and Robert J. Spinner, 319–50. Cambridge, MA: Academic Press, 2015.

Greene, Melissa Fay. "30 Years Ago, Romania Deprived Thousands of Babies of Human Contact." *The Atlantic*, June 23, 2020.

Hagerty, James R. "Texas Roadhouse CEO Kent Taylor, a Business Maverick, Was Tormented by Tinnitus after Covid-19." *Wall Street Journal*, March 24, 2021.

Hasan, Maham. "What All That Touch Deprivation Is Doing to Us." *New York Times*, October 6, 2020.

Iyengar, Smriti, Kirk W. Johnson, Michael H. Ossipov, and Sheena K. Aurora. "CGRP and the Trigeminal System in Migraine." *Headache* 59, no. 5 (May 2019): 659–81.

Khan, Sabrina, Faisal Mohammad Amin, Casper Emil Christensen, Hashmat Ghanizada, Samaira Younis, Anne Christine Rye Olinger, Patrick J. H. de Koning et al. "Meningeal Contribution to Migraine Pain: A Magnetic Resonance Angiography Study." *Brain* 142, no. 1 (January 1, 2019): 93–102.

Mason, Bianca N., and Andrew F. Russo. "Vascular Contributions to Migraine: Time to Revisit?" *Frontiers in Cellular Neuroscience* 12 (2018): 233.

McGlone, Francis, Johan Wessberg, and Håkan Olausson. "Discriminative and Affective Touch: Sensing and Feeling." *Neuron* 82, no. 4 (May 21, 2014): 737–55.

Pampush, James D., and David J. Daegling. "The Enduring Puzzle of the Human Chin." *Evolutionary Anthropology* 25, no. 1 (January 2016): 20–35.

Pietsch, Bryan. "Kent Taylor, Texas Roadhouse Founder and C.E.O., Dies at 65." *New York Times*, March 21, 2021.

Porges, Stephen. "The Role of Social Engagement in Attachment and Bonding: A Phylogenetic Perspective." In *Attachment and Bonding: A New Synthesis*, edited by C. Sue Carter, Lieselotte Ahnert, K. E. Grossmann, Sarah B. Hyrdy, Michael E. Lamb, Stephen Porges, and Norbert Sachser. Cambridge, MA: MIT Press, 2005.

Purves, Dale, George J. Augustine, David Fitzpatrick, Lawrence C. Katz, Anthony-Samuel LaMantia, James O. McNamara, and S. Mark Williams, eds. "The Blood Supply of the Brain and Spinal Cord." In *Neuroscience*. 2nd ed. Sunderland, MA: Sinauer Associates, 2001.

Robbins, Matthew S., Carrie E. Robertson, Eugene Kaplan, Jessica Ailani, Larry Charleston IV, Deena Kuruvilla, Andrew Blumenfield et al. "The Sphenopalatine Ganglion: Anatomy, Pathophysiology and Therapeutic Targeting in Headache." *Headache* 56, no. 2 (February 2016): 240–58.

Robinson, Jennifer L., Pamela M. Johnson, Karolina Kister, Michael T. Yin, Jing Chen, and Sunil Wadhwa. "Estrogen Signaling Impacts Temporomandibular Joint and Periodontal Disease Pathology." *Odontology* 108, no. 2 (April 2020): 153–65.

Roelofs, Karin. "Freeze for Action: Neurobiological Mechanisms in Animal and Human Freezing." *Philosophical Transactions of the Royal Society B* 372, no. 1718 (April 2017).

Ruff, Christopher, Brigitte Holt, and Erik Trinkaus. "Who's Afraid of the Big Bad Wolff?: 'Wolff's Law' and Bone Functional Adaptation." *American Journal of Physical Anthropology* 129, no. 4 (April 2006): 484–98.

Sangalang, Cindy C., and Cindy Vang. "Intergenerational Trauma in the Refugee Families: A Systematic Review." *Journal of Immigrant and Minority Health* 19, no. 3 (June 2017): 745–54.

Tomaszewski, Krzysztof A., Matthew J. Graves, Brandon Michael Henry, Patrick Popieluszko, Joyeeta Roy, Przemyslaw A Pekala, Wan Chin Hsieh et al. "A Surgical Anatomy of the Sciatic Nerve: A Meta-Analysis." *Journal of Orthopaedic Research* 34, no. 10 (October 2016): 1820–27.

Université Laval. "Preemies' Brains Reap Long-Term Benefits from Kangaroo Mother Care." *ScienceDaily*, 19 September 2012, www.sciencedaily.com/releases/2012/09/120919125600.htm.

Weir, Kirsten. "The Lasting Impact of Neglect." *American Psychological Association* 45, no. 6 (June 2014): 36.

Wroe, Stephen, Toni L. Ferrara, Colin R. McHenry, Darren Curnoe, and Uphar Chamoli. "The Craniomandibular Mechanics of Being Human." *Proceedings of the Royal Society B* 277, no. 1700 (December 7, 2010): 3579–86.

Yadav, Sumit, Yun Yang, Eliane H. Dutra, Jennifer L. Robinson, and Sunil Wadhwa. "Temporomandibular Joint Disorders in Older Adults." *Journal of American Geriatric Society* 66, no. 6 (2018): 1213–17.

Books

Anatomy and Physiology References

Calais-Germain, Blandine. *Anatomy of Movement*. Seattle, WA: Eastland Press, 1984.

Fonder, Aelred C., *Dental Distress Syndrome*. Chicago: Medical-Dental Arts, 1990.

Haines, Steve. *Pain Is Really Strange*. London: Singing Dragon Press, 2015.

Ide, Yoshinobu, and K. Nakazawa. *Anatomical Atlas of the Temporomandibular Joint*. Batavia, IL: Quintessence Publishing, 1991.

Kahn, Sandra, and Paul R. Ehrlich. *Jaws: The Story of a Hidden Epidemic*. Palo Alto, CA: Stanford University Press, 2018.

Keleman, Stanley. *Emotional Anatomy*. Berkeley, CA: Center Press, 1985.

Koch, Liz. *Stalking Wild Psoas*. Berkeley, CA: North Atlantic Books, 2019.

Mees, L. F. C. *Secrets of the Skeleton*. Hudson, NY: Anthroposophic Press, 1998.

Myers, Thomas W. *Anatomy Trains: Myofascial Meridians for Manual and Movement Therapists*. London: Churchill Livingstone, 2001.

Netter, Frank H. *Atlas of Human Anatomy*. 2nd ed. London: Elsevier, 1997.

Netter, Frank H. *Atlas of Human Anatomy*. 5th ed. London: Elsevier, 2010.

———. *The Ciba Collection of Medical Illustrations*, Vol. 1, *Nervous System*. Summit, NJ: Ciba Pharmaceutical, 1953.

Norton, Neil S. *Netter's Head and Neck Anatomy for Dentistry*. London: Elsevier, 2011.

Price, Weston A. *Nutrition and Physical Degeneration*. Lemon Grove, CA: Price-Pottenger, 1939.

Schultz, R. Louis, and Rosemary Feitis. *The Endless Web: Fascial Anatomy and Physical Reality*. New York: Penguin Random House, 1996.

Wilson-Pauwels, Linda. *Cranial Nerves in Health and Disease*. 2nd ed. Shelton, CT: People's Medical Publishing House, 2002.

Craniosacral, Bodywork, and Conscious Touch

Becker, Rollin E., *Life in Motion*. Portland, OR: Stillness Press, 1997.

———. *Stillness in Life*. Portland, OR: Stillness Press, 2000.

Feely, Richard, ed. *Clinical Cranial Osteopathy*. Leawood, KS: Osteopathic Cranial Academy, 1988.

Field, Tiffany. *Touch*. Cambridge, MA: MIT Press, 2003.

Frymann, Viola M. *The Collected Papers of Viola M. Frymann: Legacy of Osteopathy to Children*. Indianapolis, IN: American Academy of Osteopathy, 1998.

Haines, Steve. *Touch Is Really Strange*. London: Singing Dragon Press, 2021.

Kern, Michael. *Wisdom in the Body: The Craniosacral Approach to Essential Health.* Berkeley, CA: North Atlantic Books, 2005.

Linden, David J. *Touch: The Science of Hand, Heart, and Mind.* New York: Viking, 2015.

Magoun, Harold Ives. *Osteopathy in the Cranial Field.* Kirksville, MO: Osteopathic Cranial Association, 1951.

Milne, Hugh. *The Heart of Listening.* 2 vols. Berkeley, CA: North Atlantic Books, 1998.

Peirsmann, Etienne. *Craniosacral Therapy for Babies and Small Children.* New York: Penguin Random House, 2006.

Sills, Franklyn. *Craniosacral Biodynamics.* 2 vols. Berkeley, CA: North Atlantic Books, 2000–2004.

——. *Foundations in Craniosacral Biodynamics* 2 vols. Berkeley, CA: North Atlantic Books, 2001–2012.

——. *The Polarity Process: Energy as a Healing Art.* London: Penguin Random House, 1989.

Sumner, Ged, and Steve Haines. *Cranial Intelligence.* London: Singing Dragon Press, 2010.

Sutherland, Adah Strand. *With Thinking Fingers: The Story of William Garner Sutherland.* Leawood, KS: Osteopathic Cranial Academy, 1962.

Sutherland, William Garner. *Contributions of Thought: A Collected Writings of William Garner Sutherland.* Portland, OR: Rudra Press, 1997.

——. *The Cranial Bowl.* Leawood, KS: Osteopathic Cranial Academy, 1939.

——. *Teachings in the Science of Osteopathy.* Portland, OR: Sutherland Cranial Teaching Foundation, 2003.

Mindfulness and Loving-Kindness

Goldstein, Joseph. *A Heart Full of Peace.* Somerville, MA: Wisdom Publications, 2007.

Hanh, Thich Nhat. *Being Peace.* Berkeley, CA: Parallax Press, 1987.

——. *Peace Is Every Step.* Berkeley, CA: Parallax Press, 1990.

——. *The Sun My Heart.* Berkeley, CA: Parallax Press, 1982.

Kabat-Zinn, Jon. *Full Catastrophe Living.* New York: Penguin Random House, 1990.

——. *Wherever You Go, There You Are.* New York: Hachette Books, 1994.

Kornfield, Jack. *The Art of Forgiveness, Lovingkindness and Peace.* New York: Penguin Random House, 2002.

Levine, Stephen. *Guided Meditations, Explorations and Healings.* New York: Anchor, 1991.

Mingyur, Yongey, Rinpoche. *Joyful Wisdom: Embracing Change and Finding Freedom.* New York: Harmony Books, 2009.

——. *The Joy of Living: Unlocking the Secret and Science of Living.* New York: Three Rivers Press, 2007.

Salzberg, Sharon. *A Heart as Wide as the World: Stories on the Path of Lovingkindness.* Boston: Shambhala, 1997.

——. *The Kindness Handbook: A Practical Companion.* Louisville, CO: Sounds True, 2008.

——. *Loving Kindness: The Revolutionary Art of Happiness.* Boston: Shambhala, 1995.

Stress and Trauma

Coates, Ta-Nehisi. *Between the World and Me.* New York: Speigel and Grau, 2015.

Dana, Deb. *Polyvagal Flip Chart: Understanding the Science of Safety.* New York: W. W. Norton, 2019.

Haines, Steve. *Anxiety Is Really Strange.* London: Singing Dragon Press, 2015.

————. *Trauma Is Really Strange*. London: Singing Dragon Press, 2015.

McGonigal, Kelly. *The Upside of Stress*. New York: Penguin Random House, 2016.

Menakem, Resmaa. *My Grandmother's Hands*. Las Vegas, NV: Central Recovery Press, 2017.

Porges, Stephen. *The Pocket Guide to the Polyvagal Theory: The Transformative Power of Feeling Safe*. New York: W. W. Norton, 2017.

van der Kolk, Bessel. *The Body Keeps the Score: Brain, Mind and Body in Healing*. New York: Penguin Publishing Group, 2015.

Yoga, Ayurveda, Pranayama, and Movement Practice

Donden, Yeshi. *Health through Balance: An Introduction to Tibetan Medicine*. Translated by Jeffrey Hopkins. Ithaca, NY: Snow Lion Publications, 1986.

Donden, Yeshi, and Jhampa Kelsang. *Healing from the Source: The Science and Lore of Tibetan Medicine*. Ithaca, NY: Snow Lion Publications, 2000.

Frawley, David. *Yoga and Ayurveda: Self-Healing and Self-Realization*. Detroit, MI: Lotus Press 1999.

Koch, Liz. *Core Awareness*. Berkeley, CA: North Atlantic Books, 2012.

Lad, Vasant. *Textbook of Ayurveda Fundamental Principles*. Albuquerque, NM: Ayurvedic Press, 2002.

Lasater, Judith Hanson. *Relax and Renew: Restful Yoga for Stressful Times*. Berkeley, CA: Rodmell Press, 2011.

————. *Yogabody: Anatomy, Kinesiology and Asana*. Berkeley, CA: Rodmell Press, 2009.

Mehta, Silva, Mira Mehta, and Shyam Mehta. *Yoga the Iyengar Way*. London: Dorling Kindersley, 1990.

Miller, Elise Browning. *Yoga for Back Care*. Self-published.

————. *Yoga for Scoliosis*. Self-published, 2003.

Miller, Elise Browning, and Nancy Heraty. *Yoga for Scoliosis—a Path for Students and Teachers*. Self-published, 2016.

Moyer, Donald. *Yoga: Awakening the Inner Body*. Berkeley, CA: Rodmell Press, 1993.

————. *Yoga for Healthy Feet*. Berkeley, CA: Rodmell Press, 2016.

Nestor, James. *Breath*. New York: Riverhead Books, 2021.

Rama, Swami. *Exercises for Joints and Glands: Simple Movements to Enhance Your Well-Being*. Honesdale, PA: Himalayan Institute Press, 2007.

Scaravelli, Vanda. *Awakening the Spine: Yoga for Health, Vitality and Energy*. New York: HarperOne, 2015.

Spence, Joanne. *Trauma-Informed Yoga: A Toolbox for Therapists: 47 Simple Practices to Calm, Balance, and Restore the Nervous System*. Eau Claire, WI: PESI Publishing and Media, 2021.

Movies

Marder, Darius, dir. *The Sound of Metal*. Culver City, CA: Amazon Studios, 2020.

Podcasts

Drabble, Freddy. "Polyvagal Theory Explained with Stephen Porges, PhD," May 31, 2021, episode 5, *Chasing Consciousness*, podcast, https://www.chasingconsciousness.net/episodes.

Halford, Ryan. *The Craniosacral Podcast*. https://www.craniosacralpodcast.com/.

Seigel, Robert. "Why Do Humans Have Chins? A Scientist Explains the 'Enduring Puzzle,'" *All Things Considered*, NPR, January 29, 2016, https://www.npr.org/2016/01/29/464893281 /why-do-humans-have-chins-a-scientist-explains-the-enduring-puzzle.

Websites

Jealous, James, *lecture series*. https://traditionalosteopathyedu.com/lecture-series.

Migraine Research Foundation. https://migraineresearchfoundation.org.

Franklyn Sills. https://www.craniosacral-biodynamics.org.

Credits

Vayus and Chakras and The Tidal Body illustrated by Ronja Ver.

Excerpt from *Open Secret: Versions of Rumi* translated by Coleman Barks and John Mayne, © 1999. Reprinted by arrangement with Shambhala Publications, Inc., Boulder, CO. www.shambhala.com.

"Taking Care" by Callista Buchen, © 2019. Reprinted with permission from Black Lawrence Press.

Forgiveness Meditation by Stephen Levine reprinted with permission from Penguin Random House.

Figure 2.7: Social Engagement System is reprinted with permission from W. W. Norton & Company.

Figs. 1.1–2.6, 2.8a–2.9b, and 3.3–7.2 adapted with permission from *Craniosacral Biodynamics, Volume One: The Breath of Life, Biodynamics, and Fundamental Skills, Revised Edition* by Franklyn Sills, published by North Atlantic Books, copyright © 2001 by Franklyn Sills; *Foundations in Craniosacral Biodynamics, Volume One: The Breath of Life and Fundamental Skills* by Franklyn Sills, published by North Atlantic Books, copyright © 2011 by Franklyn Sills; and *Foundations in Craniosacral Biodynamics, Volume Two: The Sentient Embryo, Tissue Intelligence, and Trauma Resolution* by Franklyn Sills, published by North Atlantic Books, copyright © 2012 by Franklyn Sills. Reprinted by permission of publisher.

Index

addiction, 190–91

Ajahn Pasanno, 38

Allione, Tsultrim; *Women of Wisdom*, 199

animals

  lessons from, 68, 70–71

  loving-kindness for, 203

anxiety, 235, 236

  body scanning for, 219

  breathing and, 83

  effects of, 21, 61

  mindfulness of, 110, 189, 209, 239

  three questions for working with,
    237–39

  trauma and, 72–74

Aquinas, Thomas, 200

attention deficit disorder (ADD), 88, 90

Ayurveda, 39, 41, 91, 95, 114

beginner's mind, 185–86, 189

biofeedback, 103, 192

birthing, xxi, 5, 19, 53, 57, 79

body, 97

  awareness, exercises for, 141–42

  cause and effect in, 140

  direct experience of, 31

  and emotions, connection of, 110, 212,
    213, 234

  intelligence of, 93

  and jaw, interconnectedness of, xix–xx,
    42–43, 94

  listening to, 190–92

  and mind, relationship of, 12, 32, 35, 71, 72

  mindfulness of, 66–67, 219

  perfectly imbalanced, 111, 152

  right-left balance, 89–90, 91, 95, 96–97,
    138

  stabilizing and giving sides, 114

body map

  instructions, 115–18

  in Mirror Exercise, 208, 210

  purpose, 114–15, 190

  revisiting, 122, 124, 133, 139

Body Scan Meditation, 66, 124, 195

  instructions, 219–23

  when to do, 66, 232, 236, 239

body-mind, 21, 67, 72, 192

Borysenko, Joan, 229

brain

  chronic jaw tension and, 43

  development, 20

  falx and tentorium membranes, 87–88

  healthy jaw and, 21

  meninges protecting, 57, 75

  migraines and, 75

  right-left imbalances in, 96

  tidal fluctuations in, 42

  touch needed for development, 99–100

"brain breath," 39–42

brain stem, 68–69, 75

breathing

  anxiety and, 237–39

  with breath awareness, 194–95, 216–19,
    232, 237, 239

  emotions and, 234

  health and, 83

  and inner tide, relationship of, 33–34, 35

overview, 192–93, 207–8
when to do, 122, 123, 152
moon journals, 219
building library of experience in, 102, 115
intention of, 118–19, 241
migraines and, 80
resources for, 241–42
Moyer, Donald, 163

neck, xxi, 23, 27–30, 38
awareness of, 222–23
in core actions, 125, 129, 131, 137, 139
dentistry and, 6, 48
foot pain and, 93–94
headaches and, 65, 66–67, 72, 75–76
hips and, 86
in inversions, 180
jaw tension and, 48–51, 59
sinus infections and, 60
upper, 19, 60, 63
in yoga poses, 92, 123, 144, 146, 149, 153, 155, 158, 163, 166, 169, 171, 176
nervous system, 73, 217
femur rotation and, 134
formation of, 91
healthy jaw and, 21
impact of accidents on, 72
others', coregulation with, 69–70
trauma and, 68–69
See also parasympathetic nervous system; sympathetic nervous system
Netter's Head and Neck Anatomy for Dentists, 3
night guards, 5–6
Nonviolent Communication, 199, 239

obsessive-compulsive disorder (OCD), 88
occiput, 50, 60, 78, 79, 80, 87

pain
in body mapping, 117–18, 133
body scanning for, 219
chronic, 52, 66, 229, 231–32
in femur rotation, 136
foot, 92–93
jaw tension and, xxi, 3–4, 9, 21, 83 (*see also* TMD)
knee, 51–52, 139
in Lion Face Pose, 124

messages from, 64
mindfulness of, 189, 229–31
origin of, finding, 114–15
receptivity toward, 74
right/left body balance and, 111
sacrum and, 84–85
from sternocleidomastoid, 28
touch and, 99–100
in trauma release, 59–60
in yoga poses, 179
parasympathetic nervous system, 70, 71, 174, 217
Patel, Ramanand, 37, 38, 133, 139
patience, 72, 118, 125, 232
pelvic floor, 26, 85, 136, 137
pelvis, 133, 138, 151, 173
polyvagal theory, 68–69
Porges, Stephen, 20, 61, 68–69
post-traumatic stress disorder (PTSD), 21
posture
core actions and, 112, 113–14
defensive, 29
"stress," 124
trapezius overuse and, 30
prana, 33, 39. *See also* vayus ("winds")
present moment, 31, 235, 236
primitive streak, 91
proprioception, 131

reciprocal tension membrane (RTM), 56–57, 80, 88–89, 91, 96
reflexology, 94
Relaxation Response (Herbert Benson), 217
root canals, 47
Rosenberg, Marshall, 199, 239
Rumi, 26

sacrum
femur rotation and, 138
foot pain and, 93
movement of, 55–56, 58
releasing, 86–87
role of, 84
in yoga poses, 156, 158–59
safe touch, 72. *See also* conscious touch
safety, 27, 61, 69–70
Salzberg, Sharon, 191, 197
Savasana, 66
sciatica, 26, 84–85

scoliosis, 26–27, 76, 116

self-awareness, xix, xx, xxii, 103, 110, 113, 209

shoulder blades
  core actions for, 124–32, 148, 152, 153, 155,
    157–58, 160, 161–62, 165, 167
  in inversions, 168–71, 172

Shunryu Suzuki, 186

sinuses and sinusitis, 16, 40, 46–47, 59, 60,
  179

skull, pliability of, 35–36, 41

sleep apnea, 16

social engagement system, 20–21, 69–70

Sound of Metal (film), 62

sphenoid bone, 19, 24, 25, 26, 63, 76, 87

spine
  atlas and axis vertebrae, 49–50
  femur rotation and, 138
  pelvic bones and, 55
  in yoga poses, 150, 151

sternocleidomastoid muscles (SCMs),
  27–28, 66, 75

stomatognathic system, 9

stress
  causes, 77
  clenching and, 68
  in daily life, 60
  genetic markers for, 92
  in headaches, role of, 67
  Porges's definition, 69
  reduction, 109–10, 118
  relationship to, changing, 103, 192
  self-awareness and, xxii
  TMD and, 4

suicide, 61–62

Sutherland, William
  on core link, 86
  on inner tide, 133
  Iyengar yoga and, 38–39
  on reciprocal tension, 88
  role of, xx, 36–37, 41
  Sutherland's Grip, 76
  on thinking fingers, 100

sympathetic nervous system, 21, 70, 71, 174,
  213, 217. *See also* fight-or-flight response

Taking Care (Callista Buchen), 232

Taylor, Kent, 61–62

teeth, 14, 16, 23
  in facial self-massage, 103

functions of, 9, 68
  in Oral Cavity Meditation, 193, 210–12
  TMD and, xxi, 4, 5–6, 45
  in yoga poses, 123, 124, 161, 162
  See also dental work

temporalis muscle, 24–25
  blocked, 58
  dural tube and, 87
  headaches and, 65–66
  sinus infections and, 60
  tightness in, 57
  touch and, 103, 106
  vertigo and, 63

Tenzin Gyatso, Fourteenth Dalai Lama, 197

Three-Part Breathing, 136
  anxiety and, 239
  benefits, 92
  instructions, 214–15
  Lion Face and, 124
  overview, 193–94, 212–14
  in Savasana, 174, 177

tides, 32–33. *See also* inner tide

tinnitus, 59, 60, 61–62

Titmus, Christopher, 229

TMD
  breathing and, 83
  causes and repercussions, xxi, 45
  conditions linked to, 4–5, 7, 42–43, 50, 83
  hypermobility and, 96
  statistics on sufferers, 3–4
  symptom migration from, 47–51
  tracking, 102–3

TMJ
  in alignment, 9, 22
  core actions for, 122–24, 148–49, 151, 153,
    156, 158, 161, 162, 168, 170, 173
  defining, 3
  ears and, 53
  evolutionary design, 9
  feet and, 139
  lateral pterygoid and, 25–26
  misalignment and compression, 45–46
  movements, 22
  role of, 20–21
  true axis of, 48

TMJ Handbook, overview, xxi–xxii, 97–98

touch, 54, 70, 99–100. *See also* conscious
  touch

trapezius muscle, 28–30, 48, 51, 124

trauma, xxi, 54
  childhood, 70–72, 76, 84–85
  chronic pain and, 232
  dissociation from, 71, 72
  intergenerational, 91–92
  memories of, 73–74
  pain in unraveling, 59–60
  responses, 62, 70, 71
  role of, 68–69
  systemic, 5
  TMD and, xxi, 4
  touch and, 100

unwinding, 93

van der Kolk, Bessel, 48
vayus ("winds")
  apana, 39–40
  prana, 39–40 (*see also* "brain breath")
  samana, 40–41
  udana, 39–40, 41
  vyana, 40–41
vertigo, 19, 53, 62, 63–64
vision, 26, 30

whiplash, 19, 29, 51, 62–63, 93–94
wisdom tooth extraction, 46
Wolff's law, 12, 14, 16, 55
women
  migraines and, 75, 76–77
  TMD and, 3

yin and yang, 96–97
yoga, 31–32, 236
  actions and movements, distinguishing,
    112

benefits of, 109–10
central axis in, 91, 92
effort in, 112–13
general guidance, 143, 179
inversions, guidance on, 165–66, 179–80
for jaw tension, unique approach, 110–11,
  113–14
life force in, 33
long tide and, 35
See also Iyengar yoga
Yoga for Jaw Tensions workshops, xxi
yoga poses
  Bridge, 163–65
  Cat/Dog, 143–44
  Child's, 145–46
  Corpse, 174, 176–77
  Downward Dog, 146–47
  Elbow Balance, 171–73
  Half Handstand, 166–68
  Half Moon, 156–59
  Handstand, 168–71
  Puppy, 145
  Reclining Bound Angle, 174–76
  Side Angle, 154–56
  Standing Mountain, 147–49
  Warrior 2, 152–54
  Wide Leg, 149–52
  Wide Leg Forward Bend, 159–63
  See also Lion Face Pose
yoga sequences
  extended and full, 181
  limited, 180

About the Author

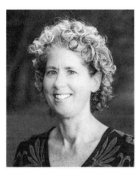

CATOR SHACHOY began the practices of yoga, meditation, and energy healing as an exploration to heal chronic illness. Her first introduction to yoga and Buddhist meditation resulted in an instant sense of reconnection—she felt at home. A similar experience occurred when exposed to energy healing. Since 1990, Cator has focused her life on continued study and training in these areas. She lived in Buddhist monasteries and spiritual communities for three years as a young adult.

Cator is a certified International Association of Yoga Therapy (C-IAYT) yoga therapist, Mindfulness Based Stress Reduction (MBSR) mindfulness instructor, and Visionary Craniosacral Work (VCSW) craniosacral practitioner. She has additional cranial training in pediatrics with Benjamin Shield and Biodynamics with Michael Shea. Cator completed teacher training at Kripalu Yoga Center and the Iyengar Yoga Institute of San Francisco and has studied with senior Iyengar teachers for over twenty years, including working closely with Ramanand Patel for a decade followed by ten years of weekly classes with Donald Moyer. Other influences include Patricia Sullivan, Judith Lasater, Elise Miller, and Mary Lou Weprin. Her movement training includes chi kung and tai chi (yin and yang styles) as well as improvisational and social dance forms. She has extensive training in the Thai forest tradition of meditation and has spent a cumulative total of several years in silent retreat. Her primary teachers include Ajahn Pasanno, Ruth Denison, and Mingyur Rinpoche.

Cator has an inclusive family-based private practice in the San Francisco

Bay area and offers therapeutic classes in Buddhism, craniosacral, mindfulness, meditation, and yoga in-person and online. She has taught for over twenty years in the United States and internationally.

For Cator, exploring yoga, meditation and craniosacral is an ever-deepening investigation into the nature of being human and alive. She wishes to support people on their journey of healing toward a more peaceful life.